W9-CHH-667

COMPACT *Research*

Chronic Fatigue Syndrome

Diseases and Disorders

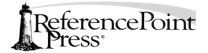

ReferencePoint
Press®

San Diego, CA

Other books in the Compact Research Diseases and Disorders set:

Acne and Skin Disorders
Fetal Alcohol Disorders
Food-Borne Illnesses
HPV
Post-Traumatic Stress Disorder

*For a complete list of titles please visit www.referencepointpress.com.

COMPACT *Research*

Chronic Fatigue Syndrome

Peggy J. Parks

Diseases and Disorders

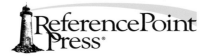

ReferencePoint Press®

San Diego, CA

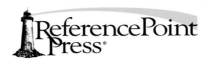

© 2012 ReferencePoint Press, Inc.
Printed in the United States

For more information, contact:
ReferencePoint Press, Inc.
PO Box 27779
San Diego, CA 92198
www.ReferencePointPress.com

Picture credits:
Cover: Dreamstime and iStockphoto.com
Maury Aaseng: 32–35, 47–49, 61–64, 76–77
David Parker/Science Photo Library: 18
Thinkstock/Comstock: 12

LIBRARY OF CONGRESS CATALOGING-IN-PUBLICATION DATA

Parks, Peggy J., 1951–
    Chronic fatigue syndrome / by Peggy J. Parks.
        p. cm. — (Compact research series)
    Includes bibliographical references and index.
    ISBN-13: 978-1-60152-228-3 (hardback)
    ISBN-10: 1-60152-228-2 (hardback)
    1. Chronic fatigue syndrome—Popular works. I. Title.
    RB150.F37P37   2012
    616'.0478—dc23
                                                    2011028505

Contents

Foreword

"Where is the knowledge we have lost in information?"

—T.S. Eliot, "The Rock."

As modern civilization continues to evolve, its ability to create, store, distribute, and access information expands exponentially. The explosion of information from all media continues to increase at a phenomenal rate. By 2020 some experts predict the worldwide information base will double every 73 days. While access to diverse sources of information and perspectives is paramount to any democratic society, information alone cannot help people gain knowledge and understanding. Information must be organized and presented clearly and succinctly in order to be understood. The challenge in the digital age becomes not the creation of information, but how best to sort, organize, enhance, and present information.

ReferencePoint Press developed the *Compact Research* series with this challenge of the information age in mind. More than any other subject area today, researching current issues can yield vast, diverse, and unqualified information that can be intimidating and overwhelming for even the most advanced and motivated researcher. The *Compact Research* series offers a compact, relevant, intelligent, and conveniently organized collection of information covering a variety of current topics ranging from illegal immigration and deforestation to diseases such as anorexia and meningitis.

The series focuses on three types of information: objective single-author narratives, opinion-based primary source quotations, and facts and statistics. The clearly written objective narratives provide context and reliable background information. Primary source quotes are carefully selected and cited, exposing the reader to differing points of view. And facts and statistics sections aid the reader in evaluating perspectives. Presenting these key types of information creates a richer, more balanced learning experience.

For better understanding and convenience, the series enhances information by organizing it into narrower topics and adding design features that make it easy for a reader to identify desired content. For example, in *Compact Research: Illegal Immigration*, a chapter covering the economic impact of illegal immigration has an objective narrative explaining the various ways the economy is impacted, a balanced section of numerous primary source quotes on the topic, followed by facts and full-color illustrations to encourage evaluation of contrasting perspectives.

The ancient Roman philosopher Lucius Annaeus Seneca wrote, "It is quality rather than quantity that matters." More than just a collection of content, the *Compact Research* series is simply committed to creating, finding, organizing, and presenting the most relevant and appropriate amount of information on a current topic in a user-friendly style that invites, intrigues, and fosters understanding.

Chronic Fatigue Syndrome at a Glance

The Illness Defined

Chronic fatigue syndrome (CFS) is characterized by extreme exhaustion that does not improve with rest or sleep and lingers for months—or even years—without relief.

Symptoms

The most common symptom of CFS is incapacitating fatigue. Other symptoms include pain, sensitivity to light and sound, and cognitive difficulties.

Prevalence

According to the Centers for Disease Control and Prevention (CDC), as many as 4 million Americans suffer from CFS. The National Institutes of Health states that the worldwide estimate is approximately 17 million.

CFS Patient Profile

People of all ages and walks of life can develop CFS, although it is much more common in adults than children or adolescents and more prevalent among women than men.

Suspected Causes

The cause of CFS is unknown. Scientific theories include viral infections, immune system dysfunction, allergies, and hormonal imbalances.

Diagnosing CFS

In the absence of specific tests to detect CFS in the body, it can only be diagnosed when all other diseases and disorders have been ruled out. According to the CDC, only about 20 percent of CFS sufferers are ever diagnosed.

Effects on Sufferers

The effects of CFS vary greatly, with some people feeling unwell much of the time but able to go about their daily lives, and others who are totally disabled and bedridden.

Treatment Options

Although no treatment specifically for CFS has been developed, physicians often prescribe medications to treat symptoms such as pain and inability to sleep. Research has shown that physical therapy combined with psychotherapy has helped some patients immensely.

Overcoming Chronic Fatigue Syndrome

No comprehensive recovery statistics exist for CFS because the majority of patients never seek treatment.

Overview

❝As the name *chronic fatigue syndrome* suggests, this illness is accompanied by fatigue. However, it's not the kind of fatigue we experience after a particularly busy day or week, after a sleepless night or after a single stressful event. It's a severe, incapacitating fatigue.❞

—The CDC, a government agency dedicated to protecting health and promoting quality of life through the prevention and control of disease, injury, and disability.

❝There has been substantial mystery surrounding the origins of Chronic Fatigue Syndrome (CFS)—a condition affecting as many as four million Americans and marked by symptoms that include a sense of weariness that sleep does not improve and difficulty with memory and concentration.❞

—Christopher Fisher, who holds a PhD in clinical health psychology and behavioral medicine and is managing editor of the online medical and psychology publication *Behavioral Medicine Report*.

Molly Billings is an attractive, intelligent 21-year-old woman who has a variety of interests. She is outgoing and social, enjoys talking to people, and prides herself on being able to carry on a conversation with most anyone. She is interested in politics, religion, and culture. Because of her fascination with the world around her, she would love to travel, but that is not possible. Billings suffers from an illness known as chronic fatigue syndrome, so most of her time is spent at home. "Sometimes I feel like I have more in common with my grandparents than my peers," she says. "I have difficulty sleeping. I'm usually sore . . . my head constantly hurts, I'm sensitive to light, sound, and particular smells, and I tire in doing the simplest tasks. I always feel worn out and tired. Sometimes I feel like I'm a twenty-one year old woman stuck in a body that feels eighty."[1]

Billings was a freshman in high school when she first became ill, and for the next three years she was bedridden. During her senior year she was confined to a wheelchair and had to be physically posed for her senior pictures. The specialists she saw did not take her illness seriously and accused her of faking her symptoms

> **CFS is a complex illness that results in severe fatigue to the point of being incapacitating.**

to get attention. She writes: "Most physicians dismiss patients who have this particular illness as crazies, or at best, people who are in need of mental care. I'm sure they believe that most people who claim to be sick are hypochondriacs, lazy, or are people desperately seeking attention." Billings adds that while this might be true in some cases, "on behalf of all the patients who actually are sick, I can tell you this is usually a horrendous falsehood."[2]

What Is Chronic Fatigue Syndrome?

CFS is a complex illness that results in severe fatigue to the point of being incapacitating. It has been called many different names over the years as researchers and physicians have struggled to figure out what it is. The current name was designated by the CDC in 1988, but the illness is also referred to as *chronic fatigue and immune dysfunction syndrome* (CFIDS) and *myalgic encephalomyelitis* (ME), which is the common term in Canada, Australia, and European countries.

CFS is recognized by the CDC and other health organizations as a physical disorder with symptoms that range from flu-like discomfort to total incapacitation. Many medical professionals, however, remain skeptical that CFS is an actual illness. Rather, they believe that it is a purely psychological phenomenon, an imaginary ailment from which patients could recover if they wanted to badly enough. CFS sufferers and advocacy organizations attribute much of this skepticism to the name itself.

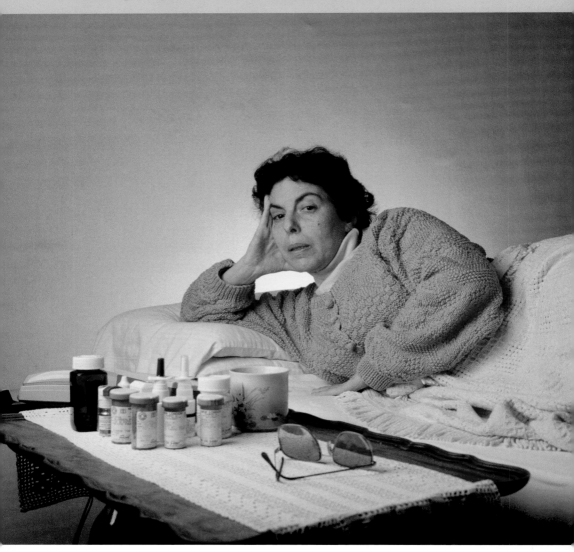

Chronic fatigue syndrome, which is characterized by extreme exhaustion that does not improve with rest or sleep and lingers for months or even years, is more prevalent in women than in men. Symptoms of the disorder include pain, sensitivity to light and sound, and cognitive difficulties.

This is the perspective of Laura Hillenbrand, the author of the books *Seabiscuit* and *Unbroken*, who has suffered from severe CFS since she was 19 years old. She explains: "It's exasperating because of the name, which is condescending and so grossly misleading. Fatigue is what we experience, but it is what a match is to an atomic bomb."[3]

Millions of Sufferers

Although the CDC estimates that from 1 million to 4 million Americans are afflicted with CFS, the actual prevalence is unknown. Since only about 20 percent of them seek medical attention, most who suffer from the illness do not realize they have it and are never diagnosed. According to the CFIDS Association of America, an estimated 17 million people worldwide suffer from CFS, which can strike males and females both young and old and of all walks of life. The group explains: "CFS does not discriminate. It strikes people of all age, racial, ethnic and socioeconomic groups. Research has shown that it is 3–4 times more common in women compared to men, a rate similar to that of autoimmune conditions like multiple sclerosis and lupus."[4]

CFS is rare among teenagers, but the illness does sometimes affect young people. A study published in April 2011 by researchers from the Netherlands was one of the few that focused on prevalence among adolescents aged 10 to 18. After surveying Dutch physicians, the team found that only about 1 in 900 youth suffered from CFS, and the average age of onset was 15 years. Another finding was that about half of the young people experienced symptoms for at least 17 months before they were diagnosed. The researchers concluded that the condition appears to be underrecognized by primary care physicians, as an April 18, 2011, Reuters article explains: "Only half of all general practitioners who agreed to participate in the study said they accepted CFS as a distinct diagnosis, versus 96 percent of the pediatricians consulted during the study. And nearly 75 percent of teens with CFS were not diagnosed by their general practitioners."[5]

A Range of Symptoms

The symptoms of CFS vary from person to person, as the Mayo Clinic states: "People with chronic fatigue syndrome may experience a variety of signs and symptoms that come and go frequently with no identifiable pattern."[6] There are some commonalities among sufferers, though, such as extreme exhaustion that is made worse by physical or mental activity and does not improve with rest or sleep. Often those who develop CFS suffer from memory loss and concentration problems, as well as unusual pain in their joints and muscles. One of the most common complaints of people with CFS is that its onset feels like the flu, with symptoms such as headache, muscle aches, chills, sore throat, and mildly enlarged lymph nodes. The difference, however, is that CFS lingers for months—or even years—with no signs of abating and no relief for the patient.

Laurel Bertrand has suffered from CFS for 15 years, and she still remembers the exact moment when she was stricken with it: the afternoon of New Year's Eve in 1996. She was in her apartment when suddenly she felt like she "had been hit with a ton of bricks. I remember stopping in my tracks as I leaned my hand against the wall to hold myself up. 'What the heck . . . ?' I murmured out loud, astounded by how abruptly ill I felt. . . . What bad timing, I thought, to have apparently come down with the flu on New Year's Eve."[7]

> **The largest CFS outbreak ever recorded in the United States began in 1984 at Incline Village, an upscale resort town on the Nevada side of Lake Tahoe.**

As miserable as Bertrand felt, she was determined not to give in to what she thought was a simple bug, and she went ahead with her plans to celebrate with friends. But as she headed downtown on the bus, she had no doubt that something was very wrong. She writes: "As I sat in my seat, eyes closed from lights that felt too bright, I remember everyone's voices seemed simultaneously too loud and yet somehow distant and muffled, as though we were all mysteriously traveling underwater. I felt myself sweating from fever, though it was below freezing outside." Bertrand managed to get through the evening, and as midnight approached she and her friends counted down the last seconds of the year. "'10 . . . 9 . . . 8 . . .' Little did I know at the time," she says, "that I was not just counting down the last few moments of 1996, but the last few moments of my life as I had known it."[8]

CFS Clusters

Over the years a number of community-wide outbreaks of CFS have been reported. One of the first occurred during the fall and winter of 1948 to 1949 in Akureyri, a town on the northern coast of Iceland, in which nearly 500 people became sick. The epidemic was first thought to be poliomyelitis (more commonly known as polio) because the patients had become paralyzed, and paralysis is the hallmark of polio. This assumption proved to be incorrect, however, as the authors of an April 1950 article in the *American Journal of Hygiene* explained: "After the third and fourth weeks it became evident that this epidemic differed in many respects from the previously known epidemics of poliomyelitis."[9] Decades passed before the mysterious illness dubbed "Icelandic disease" was attributed to what came to be known as chronic fatigue syndrome.

> " No one is more eager to know what causes CFS than the millions of people who suffer from it—and no one is more frustrated at repeatedly being told that the cause is unknown. "

The largest CFS outbreak ever recorded in the United States began in 1984 at Incline Village, an upscale resort town on the Nevada side of Lake Tahoe. Physicians Paul R. Cheney and Daniel L. Peterson treated several groups of patients who became sick within a few months of each other, including 16 teachers and 6 students from 3 different high schools and 11 casino employees. The number of sick patients continued to grow, with nearly 300 cases of the mysterious illness reported by 1987. Their symptoms ranged from fever, headaches, and sore throats to seizures, severe memory loss, and permanent disability, with 29 percent of the patients completely bedridden.

What Causes Chronic Fatigue Syndrome?

No one is more eager to know what causes CFS than the millions of people who suffer from it—and no one is more frustrated at repeatedly being told that the cause is unknown. Even after decades of research, knowledge about the causes of CFS is limited to scientific theories rather than certainties, because scientists have not been able to find an actual cause. The CDC writes: "The cause or causes of CFS remain unknown, despite a vigorous search. While a single cause for CFS may yet be identified, another possibility is that CFS represents a common endpoint of disease resulting from multiple causes."[10] Proposed contributors to the disease, according to the CDC, include immune system dysfunction, exposure to toxic substances, allergies, nutritional deficiency, and/or abnormally low blood pressure (hypotension).

Research has also suggested that genetics plays a role in the development of CFS. According to the University of Maryland Medical Center, the disease has been linked with genetic abnormalities in the hypothalamic-pituitary-adrenal axis, which is an area in the brain that controls response to trauma, injury, and other stressful events. The group adds that studies have found alterations in genes involved with immune function, communication between cells, and transfer of energy to cells. "Researchers have identified many different genes in patients with CFS related to blood disease, immune system function, and infection. However, no clear pattern has been found."[11]

Suspicious Links to Viruses

One of the most aggressively pursued theories related to CFS is the possibility that it is caused by one or more viruses. For instance, Epstein-Barr, which is a member of the herpes virus family, causes mononucleosis, and many patients with mono have gone on to develop CFS. This was the case with Leonard A. Jason, a psychology professor and director of the Center for Community Research at DePaul University who was stricken with CFS after a bout with mono in 1990. Jason says that through his experience, he learned "just how mysterious and frustrating the illness is. I also realized how easy it is for people to confuse the experience of everyday tiredness with the incapacitating illness known as CFS."[12]

> **Only when all other diseases have been ruled out can CFS be diagnosed.**

Of particular interest to scientists is a potential link between CFS and a family of viruses known as retroviruses. Retroviruses have the ability to insert themselves into the genetic material of host cells and permanently alter their DNA—which also makes them the most dangerous viruses of all. New York physician and CFS specialist David S. Bell writes: "After the retrovirus enters the cell, it makes a DNA copy of itself and splices itself into the human chromosome. . . . There it looks and acts exactly like the human genetic material. It is no longer really a virus, an outside agent, vulnerable to the immune response. It is now human DNA. It is the perfect spy, forged or counterfeit DNA."[13] Once the virus has evolved in this way, it begins to reproduce—and as Bell explains, the immune system is powerless to stop it.

Two retroviruses are known to affect humans: HIV, which causes AIDS, and HTLV, which infects white blood cells and causes leukemia and lymphoma. A third type, xenotropic murine leukemia virus–related virus (XMRV), was discovered in 2006 when it was found in tissue samples of men with prostate cancer. Since later studies did not show such an association,

> People with CFS suffer not only from crushing fatigue, pain, and other debilitating physical problems, but also emotional anguish.

whether XMRV can cause diseases in humans is still unknown. Scientists remain interested in the retrovirus as a possible cause of CFS. At least one study suggested there might be a connection, so research continues.

A Diagnosis of Exclusion

CFS is an illness for which there is no diagnostic test, which makes diagnosis challenging. Extreme fatigue, the most obvious and consistent symptom of CFS, is present in many other illnesses. Another challenge in diagnosing CFS is that many sufferers appear to be healthy, as the CDC writes: "CFS is an invisible illness and many patients don't look sick."[14] If a patient has experienced six or more months of severe fatigue, accompanied by memory loss, generalized muscle pain (myalgia), and/or other symptoms connected to CFS, a physician will order a series of diagnostic tests to screen for infections, multiple sclerosis, tumors, or immune system disorders. Only when all other diseases have been ruled out can CFS be diagnosed.

Two difficult years passed before Laurel Bertrand was finally diagnosed with CFS. Her doctor originally thought she had mononucleosis, and he advised her to stay home and rest for at least two weeks—but months passed and she was still as sick as ever. Bertrand went through "a myriad of tests and skeptical doctors" before she was finally given the

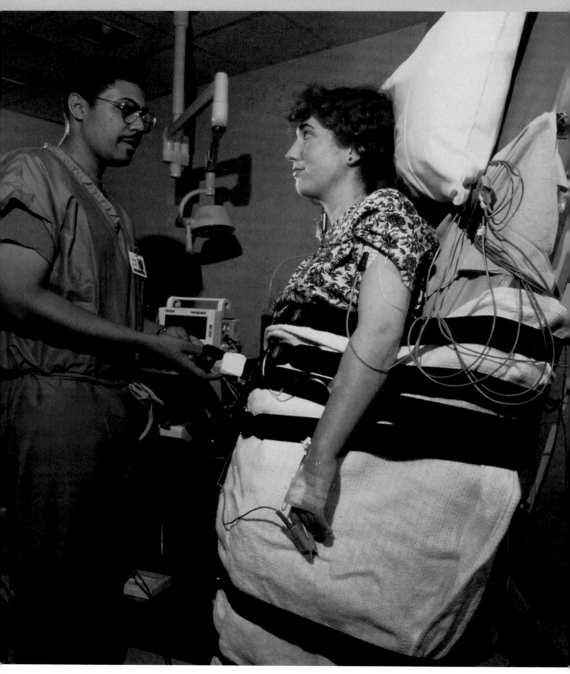

A patient prepares to undergo a diagnostic tilt table test. The test will reproduce dizziness and blackouts associated with a disorder that has been linked to chronic fatigue syndrome. Recent research suggests that treatment for the one disorder may benefit some CFS patients.

CFS diagnosis. At first, when a doctor suggested that she had CFS, she did not know what it was. She writes: "I thought he was just telling me what I already knew: that, following mono, I had become chronically ill and exhausted. It wasn't until another doctor brought it up again that I realized that was actually a name for an illness. 'I feel way too sick to have something called chronic fatigue syndrome,' I told her."[15]

What Are the Effects of Chronic Fatigue Syndrome?

The physical problems associated with CFS depend on the severity of the illness. Some patients may recover after a few months, while others do not get better and remain incapacitated. Hillary Johnson, a journalist and the author of *Osler's Web: Inside the Labyrinth of the Chronic Fatigue Syndrome Epidemic*, writes: "Many people don't realize how severe this illness can be. . . . Many patients are bedridden. And recovery is rare. A significant number of patients have been ill for more than two decades."[16]

Alexis Cairns, who has suffered from CFS for 10 years, says that one of the worst effects of the illness is the sudden "crashes" that often follow overexertion or stress. She writes: "A typical crash, for me, includes increased fatigue, mental fogginess, headaches and weird pains, achiness, and increased sensitivity to noise."[17] In November 2010 Cairns suffered a crash that severely impaired her vision. She developed extreme sensitivity to light and profound weakness of her eye muscles, which made it impossible for her to focus on anything without major discomfort. "I cannot look at anything," she says, "not words on a page, the remote control, the labels on my medication and supplement bottles, or the numbers on the phone touch pad."[18]

Emotional Trauma

People with CFS suffer not only from crushing fatigue, pain, and other debilitating physical problems, but also emotional anguish. According to the CDC, feelings of anger, guilt, anxiety, isolation, and abandonment are common among CFS patients. "While it's normal to have such feelings," the agency writes, "unresolved emotions and stress can make symptoms worse."[19]

A major part of the turmoil for CFS sufferers is the lingering skepticism over whether the disease is real or imagined. Johnson writes: "Being

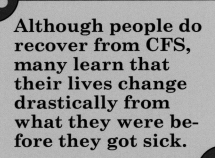

> Although people do recover from CFS, many learn that their lives change drastically from what they were before they got sick.

seriously ill for years, even decades, is nightmarish enough, but patients are also the targets of ridicule and hostility that stem from the perception that it is all in their heads."[20] Johnson refers to the 1980s CFS epidemic at Incline Village, Nevada. The CDC sent investigators to look into the outbreak, but according to Johnson, they "dismissed the epidemic and said the Tahoe doctors 'had worked themselves into a frenzy.'" Johnson says that the CFS patients were scorned and accused of faking their illness, as well as denied medical care. "Soon," she writes, "the malady came to be widely considered a personality disorder or something that sufferers brought upon themselves."[21]

Can People Overcome Chronic Fatigue Syndrome?

Since a large majority of chronic fatigue sufferers never seek medical care, their chances of overcoming the illness are poor. For those who are diagnosed, treatments are determined on an individual basis, as the Mayo Clinic states: "There's no specific chronic fatigue syndrome treatment. In general, doctors aim to relieve signs and symptoms by using a combination of treatments."[22] This combination may include daily activity moderation and gradual but steady exercise, as well as cognitive behavioral therapy to help patients work through problems and learn to manage their illness. Specific issues such as depression, pain, and sleep problems may be treated with medications.

Although people do recover from CFS, many learn that their lives change drastically from what they were before they got sick. As Billings has learned from personal experience, it may be necessary for CFS sufferers to accept that pain, intermittent fatigue, and physical limitations are things they must learn to live with. "Life is a struggle," she says. "Every moment, whether you know it or not, is a fight for survival. It's a long winding road that seemingly has no end. Sometimes it's easier than others. . . . Sometimes it's much harder. My life generally feels like the latter." Billings tries to have a positive attitude and still hopes for an eventual recovery, but she faces many hurdles. "This is something that happened to me and I have to live with it every day."[23]

Mysteries Abound

Since the first cases of CFS were reported, the illness has puzzled scientists and caused misery for those who suffer from it. Scientists have aggressively pursued studies in an effort to better understand CFS, and this has led to many potential contributors being identified—but its cause remains a mystery. As research continues, more will undoubtedly be learned, and perhaps the cause or causes will be found. For the millions of CFS sufferers throughout the world, that day cannot possibly come soon enough.

What Is Chronic Fatigue Syndrome?

> **In chronic fatigue syndrome, people are facing an energy crisis so they can only walk or exercise to a certain point, beyond which they crash and burn.**
>
> —Jacob Teitelbaum, who recovered from chronic fatigue syndrome in 1975 and is now medical director of the Fibromyalgia and Fatigue Centers.

> **A number of misconceptions and much speculation surround this mysterious disorder.**
>
> —Robert H. Shmerling, clinical chief in the Rheumatology Division at Boston's Beth Israel Deaconess Medical Center.

On May 11, 2011, investigative science reporter Mindy Kitei gave an emotional presentation at a meeting of the Chronic Fatigue Syndrome Advisory Committee in Washington, DC. Kitei has covered issues related to CFS for 20 years, and she also created a blog called *CFS Central* in honor of her friend, Nancy Kaiser, who died from CFS in June 2008. Kitei told the group: "I naively thought she'd never succumb to the illness, as if by sheer will she'd keep herself alive."[24] Formerly an avid golfer and swimmer, Kaiser had suddenly fallen ill at the age of 38 and never recovered. Eventually her eyesight failed, she had multiple seizures every day, and she was forced to crawl rather than walk because her blood pressure plummeted whenever she tried to stand or even sit up. By the time CFS claimed her life, Kaiser had seen more than 200 specialists— but not one could tell her what was wrong.

In her impassioned speech, Kitei referred to the disease as myalgic encephalomyelitis, and she had stern words for those who minimized its severity: "Despite its gravity, despite ample evidence that ME is an infectious disease, the government treats it like a joke." She admonished the CDC for focusing on "bogus psychological studies," as well as what she perceived as the agency's unwillingness to take CFS seriously enough to devote adequate resources to studying it. "To the CDC and NIH [National Institutes of Health] scientists who've been doing this ludicrous research for three decades and sweeping a worldwide human catastrophe of 17 million people under the carpet," Kitei said, "I say to you: Have you no sense of decency at long last?"[25]

A History of Mystery

No one knows exactly when the first case of CFS occurred, but the illness has been discussed in medical literature since the nineteenth century. In an April 20, 1869, article in the *Boston Medical and Surgical Journal*, American neurologist George Miller Beard referred to an affliction called neurasthenia, meaning "nervous exhaustion." He stated that the "malady" was characterized by "general malaise, debility of all the functions, poor appetite, abiding weakness in the back and spine . . . hysteria, insomnia, hypochondriases, disinclination for consecutive mental labor, severe and weakening attacks of sick headache, and other analogous symptoms." Beard explained that if these symptoms were present in a patient, but there was no evidence of any organic disease, "we have reason to suspect that the central nervous system is mainly at fault, and that we are dealing with a typical case of neurasthenia."[26]

In the years after the publication of Beard's paper, other scientists published articles about the mystifying illness and offered their own theories about it. Of particular interest were a number of

> " In an April 20, 1869, article in the *Boston Medical and Surgical Journal,* American neurologist George Miller Beard referred to an affliction called neurasthenia, meaning 'nervous exhaustion.' "

outbreaks such as one in 1955 at the Royal Free Hospital in London, England, in which nearly 300 staff members became ill. The following year the British journal the *Lancet* ran an editorial titled "A New Clinical Entity?" that discussed the London epidemic along with several others. The authors suggested the diagnostic term *benign myalgic encephalomyelitis*, with the word *benign* signifying that no one had died from the illness. The proposed name, according to the editorial, "in no way prejudices the arguments for or against a single or a related group of causal agents; and it does describe some of the striking features," including signs of damage to the brain and spinal cord, muscle pain and cramping, and partial loss of movement, as well as "a relatively benign outcome."[27]

"What's in a Name?"

Neurasthenia and *benign myalgic encephalomyelitis* are just two of many terms that have been proposed for CFS over the years. What the illness is called is extremely important to those who suffer from it, largely because they are convinced that the name has a significant impact on how it is perceived by medical professionals, as well as the general public. Karen Lee Richards, who suffers from both fibromyalgia and CFS and is the cofounder of the National Fibromyalgia Association, says this is an issue that evokes strong feelings and passionate beliefs. She writes: "The one thing just about every CFS patient agrees on, though, is that the name needs to change." Richards explains the importance of what the illness is called by using an analogy:

> More than 400 years ago in his play *Romeo and Juliet* William Shakespeare wrote, "What's in a name? That which we call a rose by any other name would smell as sweet." But I daresay if that rose were named "thorny branch" after one of its prominent characteristics, few people would bother to smell it and discover its beautiful fragrance. Unfortunately the name Chronic Fatigue Syndrome is the equivalent of thorny branch. Because CFS doesn't sound all that bad, it is difficult to get the medical community, government, and general public to look deeper and discover just how serious the illness is.[28]

To show how serious CFS sufferers are about getting rid of the *chronic fatigue syndrome* moniker, Rich Carson launched a crusade called Campaign for a Fair Name. Carson is a former long-distance runner who was stricken with CFS during the summer of 1981. Although he was devastated that life as he had known it was over, he refused to let the illness defeat him and became an activist for the CFS cause. In 2006 Carson recruited a team of eight CFS specialists to serve on an advisory board, as well as formed a Fair Name Implementation Committee, which grew to more than 20 prominent leaders from CFS research, medical, advocacy, philanthropic, and patient communities. For his work on behalf of CFS sufferers, Carson has received hundreds of letters of support, with

> **What the illness is called is extremely important to those who suffer from it, largely because they are convinced that the name has a significant impact on how it is perceived by medical professionals, as well as the general public.**

one in particular that he says stands out: "My favorite letter was from someone who said that calling this disease Chronic Fatigue Syndrome is like calling Parkinson's disease 'Chronic Shakiness Syndrome' or calling Alzheimer's disease, 'Chronic Forgetfulness Syndrome.'"[29]

The Debate over Accuracy

In general, CFS sufferers tend to favor the term *myalgic encephalomyelitis* (ME), which is used throughout Europe as well as in Australia and several other countries. Richards writes: "Although dozens of different names have been suggested to replace CFS, the discussion always seems to come back to ME. . . . It's not surprising that ME continues to rise to the top of the name-change pool. It has been used in medical literature for 50 years, which automatically gives it more familiarity and credibility in the medical community."[30] Yet not everyone agrees that *myalgic encephalomyelitis* is an appropriate name for the illness. A 1996 paper by the United Kingdom's Royal College of Physicians, Psychiatrists, and General Practitioners proposed that the term *myalgic encephalomyelitis* be dropped because it implies inflammation of the brain and central nervous system, and no such condition has ever been proved. Instead, the authors expressed their support for the diagnostic term *chronic fatigue syndrome*, which was recommended by the CDC in 1988.

One physician who rejects the diagnostic term *myalgic encephalomyelitis* is Dov Michaeli, a former biochemistry professor who founded a biotechnology firm in Larkspur, California. He writes: "Physicians who specialize in treating these patients, aided and abetted by advocacy groups, made it their mission to lend 'scientific' credibility to the condition by trying to rid it of the vague 'fatigue' term and substitute it with respectable-sounding names such as benign myalgic encephalomyelitis."[31]

> **Numerous outbreaks of mysterious fatigue-related illnesses have been reported over the years, with one of the most widely publicized occurring in a tiny farming community in upstate New York called Lyndonville.**

Michaeli emphasizes that he does not dismiss CFS, nor does he claim that it does not exist. What he objects to is the use of a diagnostic term that does not accurately define it. In reference to *myalgic encephalomyelitis* and several other names that have been proposed, such as *chronic fatigue and immune dysfunction syndrome*, *chronic infectious mononucleosis*, and *epidemic myalgic encephalomyelitis*, Michaeli writes: "Trouble is, there is not a shred of evidence for any of those. No muscle pathology, no central nervous system pathology, no immune deficiency evidence, no trace of mononucleosis. It was sheer semantic invention."[32]

Small Town, Big Problem

Numerous outbreaks of mysterious fatigue-related illnesses have been reported over the years, with one of the most widely publicized occurring in a tiny farming community in upstate New York called Lyndonville. It started during the fall of 1985, when eight children suddenly developed what appeared to be an identical illness, with symptoms such as high fever, body aches, and sore throats. Their doctor, David S. Bell, initially thought it was the flu, or perhaps mononucleosis, but he soon learned that he was dealing with something far more severe. Three weeks went by, then a month, and then six months, and still all of the children were too sick to go back to school. "I assumed they were going to get better," says Bell, "but then they never did."[33] Over the next two years, the mysterious sickness continued to spread, with 214 people (including 46 children) being stricken with it—nearly one-quarter of the town's population. More than two decades passed before the epidemic was determined to be CFS.

In the years since the Lyndonville outbreak began, Bell has stayed in close touch with his patients, and today he continues to monitor their progress. Fewer than half have fully recovered from CFS, with the rest suffering from persistent symptoms—including 20 percent who are totally disabled. Bell has devoted his career to CFS, conducting research, writing papers, giving presentations, and acting as a consultant to other physicians.

> " According to the CFIDS Association of America, thousands of servicemen and servicewomen who have returned from the current war in Iraq have suffered from multisystem illnesses, including CFS. "

In the process he has become a renowned authority on the illness, yet he makes it clear that his patients are more important than anything else. "Even though I haven't been able to remove all of their symptoms," says Bell, "I've never lost faith in those particular people. I've never given up on them, and that's the only thing that I feel really proud of."[34]

Battle Scars

In a 2009 paper published in the *Veterans Law Review*, retired Board of Veterans' Appeals chair James P. Terry discussed the various ailments that affect military personnel who have served in war zones. "One interesting aspect of the symptoms commonly associated with war-related medical and psychological illnesses," Terry writes, "is that they have been observed in each of our country's major conflicts."[35] Many of these maladies suffered by veterans are not well understood or easily defined, and are thus categorized as undiagnosed, unexplained, or multisystem illnesses. According to Terry, these illnesses involve "one or more symptoms that do not conform to a characteristic clinical presentation, or allow for a specific diagnosis, and which appear to be causing a decline in the veteran's functional status or quality of life."[36]

In reference to the servicemen and servicewomen who served in the Persian Gulf War (1990 to 1991), Terry cites one study showing that nearly 40 percent developed mild to moderate multisystem illnesses and 6 percent suffered from severe multisystem illnesses. Their symptoms included fatigue, anxiety, sleeplessness, difficulties with memory and concentration, severe joint pain, stiffness, and muscle pain. These veterans were diagnosed with a variety of ailments, including post-traumatic stress disorder, panic disorder, and CFS.

According to the CFIDS Association of America, thousands of servicemen and servicewomen who have returned from the more recent war in Iraq have suffered from multisystem illnesses, including CFS. Few studies, however, have focused exclusively on military personnel. A search of the Defense Medical Surveillance System found that more than 5,000 military personnel had been diagnosed with CFS between 1999 and 2009, as the group writes: "This is likely to be a vast underestimate, given the frequent use of other diagnostic codes for CFS symptoms, and underrecognition of CFS by military health care professionals that mirrors the low rate of diagnosis (20 percent) in the civilian population."[37]

The Puzzle Remains Unsolved

CFS has been an issue of confusion and controversy for more than a century, with even the name itself being a topic of heated debate. Scientists have aggressively pursued studies in an effort to better understand the illness, but after decades of research it still remains mysterious. Yet despite the fact that so much is unknown about CFS, and many aspects of the illness are still controversial, Bell regards the future with a positive outlook. "These are issues that must be resolved by scientists," he says. "The good news is that smart people will figure it out."[38]

What Is Chronic Fatigue Syndrome?

66 Because its symptoms are difficult to measure, CFS wasn't widely accepted as a real medical condition for several years. Today, however, doctors and researchers agree that this chronic condition should be taken seriously. 99

—Mayo Clinic, "Chronic Fatigue Syndrome," June 10, 2009. www.mayoclinic.com.

The Mayo Clinic is a world-renowned medical facility headquartered in Rochester, Minnesota.

66 It has been twenty years since chronic fatigue syndrome was recognized by major medical organizations as a legitimate medical condition. Still, there are many in the medical profession who doubt its existence. 99

—Mark Borigini, "Awakening to the Reality of Chronic Fatigue Syndrome," *Overcoming Pain* (blog), *Psychology Today*, November 18, 2009. www.psychologytoday.com.

Borigini is a physician who specializes in treating (and training others to treat) a wide variety of illnesses that cause chronic pain and disability.

Primary Source Quotes

❝Symptoms of CFS vary widely from person to person and may be serious or mild. Most symptoms cannot be seen by others, which makes it hard for friends, family members, and the public to understand the challenges a person with CFS faces.❞

—National Women's Health Information Center, "Chronic Fatigue Syndrome: Frequently Asked Questions," September 22, 2009. www.womenshealth.gov.

The National Women's Health Information Center is dedicated to improving the health and well-being of all women and girls in the United States.

❝Chronic fatigue is in part a misnomer. The syndrome often has more to do with immune system abnormalities than pervasive tiredness—although the two can go hand in hand.❞

—Katherine Harmon, "Retrovirus Linked to Chronic Fatigue Syndrome, Could Aid in Diagnosis," *Scientific American*, October 8, 2009. www.scientificamerican.com.

Harmon is a science and health writer for *Scientific American*.

❝Most people, when they hear the disease name, it's all they know about it. It sounds so mild. When I first was sick, for the first 10 years or so, I was dismissed. I was ridiculed and told I was lazy. It was a joke.❞

—Laura Hillenbrand, interviewed by Tara Parker-Pope, "An Author Escapes from Chronic Fatigue Syndrome," *Well* (blog), *New York Times,* February 4, 2011. http://well.blogs.nytimes.com.

Hillenbrand, the author of the books *Seabiscuit* and *Unbroken*, has suffered from severe CFS since she was 19 years old.

❝Now, this is not to say that CFS is not real—it probably is. But a definition based on symptoms and a long list of conditions that masquerade as CFS makes it hard to pin down with any degree of certainty.❞

—Dov Michaeli, "The Puzzle of Chronic Fatigue Syndrome," *The Doctor Weighs In* (blog), February 21, 2011. www.thedoctorweighsin.com.

Michaeli, a former professor at the University of California–San Francisco, is the founder and CEO of a biotech company located in Larkspur, California.

66 Until now, I've told no one except a small inner-circle of family that my mysterious breakdown in health, vitality, and cognition that started the night of May 5, 2007 was not due to an exotic virus I picked up in the Congo while on assignment for *National Geographic*. The truth? I'm actually a textbook case of someone with CFS, a syndrome I sniffed at until it happened to me. **99**

—John Falk, "Chronic Fatigue Syndrome and Psychotherapy," *Huffington Post*, March 1, 2011. www.huffingtonpost.com.

Falk is a journalist and author who suffered from CFS for more than three years before he told anyone about his illness.

66 Owing to the difficulty in diagnosing a chronic disorder with diffuse symptoms, many people with the disease feel they have been marginalized by the medical community—told that there is no help for them, or even that they are imagining their symptoms. **99**

—*Nature*, "Cause for Concern," editorial, March 16, 2011. www.nature.com.

Nature is a noted international weekly journal of science.

What Is Chronic Fatigue Syndrome?

- The CDC estimates that **10 to 20 times** as many people may have a condition similar to CFS that does not meet the criteria for diagnosis.

- The first recorded outbreak of CFS was at Los Angeles County Hospital in 1934, during which nearly **200 staff members** became sick.

- The Mayo Clinic states that CFS is most common among people in their **forties and fifties**, but the illness can affect people of all ages.

- According to Nancy G. Klimas, director of the University of Miami School of Medicine's Department of Immunology, only **16 percent to 17 percent** of people with CFS have been diagnosed.

- A study published in May 2011 by researchers from the Netherlands showed that the prevalence of youth CFS diagnosed by general practitioners was approximately **111 per 100,000** adolescents, with an annual incidence of **12 per 100,000**.

- According to the CFIDS Association of America, many children with CFS have what is known as **orthostatic intolerance**, which is the inability to tolerate an upright posture.

- The National Institutes of Health states that CFS most commonly affects women aged **30 to 50**.

- A July 2009 *Pediatrics* article by researchers from Chicago states that the rate of CFS is only about **0.2 percent** among adolescents.

Symptoms of Chronic Fatigue Syndrome

Chronic fatigue syndrome is characterized by extreme fatigue that often worsens with physical activity and does not improve with rest. People who suffer from this illness experience a wide range of other symptoms as well.

Primary Symptoms of CFS

Extreme exhaustion lasting more than 24 hours after physical or mental exercise

Loss of memory or concentration

Sore throat

Painful and mildly enlarged lymph nodes in the neck or armpits

Muscle pain; pain that moves from one joint to another without swelling or redness

Headache of a new type, pattern, or severity

Unrefreshing sleep

Additional CFS Symptoms

Abdominal pain

Allergies/sensitivity to foods, alcohol, odors, chemicals, medications, or noise

Visual disturbances: blurring, sensitivity to light, eye pain, dry eyes

Nausea, chills, night sweats

Irregular heartbeat, chest pain, shortness of breath

Dizziness, balance problems, fainting

Jaw pain, earache

Psychological problems; depression, irritability, anxiety disorders, panic attacks

Source: Mayo Foundation for Medical Education and Research, "Chronic Fatigue Syndrome," June 19, 2009. www.riversideonline.com.

The Name Controversy

The name "chronic fatigue syndrome" was established by the Centers for Disease Control and Prevention in 1988. Since that time, the name has been an issue of heated debate, with many sufferers and patient advocates saying that CFS trivializes the seriousness of the condition. Nearly all participants in a 2011 poll by the *Boston Globe* wanted the name changed, although they had different ideas about what it should be called.

Should Chronic Fatigue Syndrome Get a New Name?

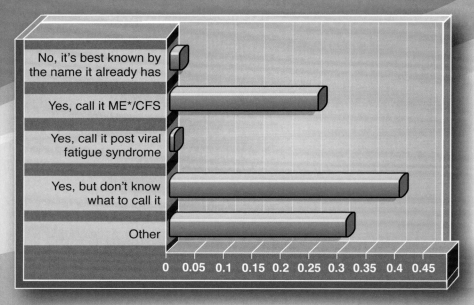

* ME = myalgic encephalomyelitis

Source: Deborah Kotz, "Does Chronic Fatigue Syndrome Deserve a Better Name?," *Boston Globe*, June 1, 2011. www.boston.com.

- According to the National Women's Health Center, although people of all income levels can develop CFS, some evidence shows that it is more common in **lower-income** than in higher-income individuals.

- The diagnostic term *myalgic encephalomyelitis* is often used in place of *chronic fatigue syndrome*; since 1969 ME has been recognized by the World Health Organization as a distinct neurological disease.

Fatigue-Related Illnesses

Since the 1930s a number of outbreaks of mysterious, fatigue-related illnesses have been reported in the United States, New Zealand, Iceland, the United Kingdom, and South Africa. Over the years some physicians and researchers have become convinced that chronic fatigue syndrome was responsible for some, and perhaps all, of the cases.

Year	Location	Number of Cases
1934	Los Angeles, California	198
1948–1949	Akureyi, Iceland	465
1950	New York State	33
1953	Rockville, Maryland	50
1955	Durban, South Africa	128
1955	London, United Kingdom	292
1956	Punta Gorda, Florida	150
1961–1962	New York State	26
1970–1971	London, United Kingdom	145
1982–1983	Tapanui, New Zealand	28
1984–1987	Incline Village, Nevada	300
1984–1987	Yates, New York	21*

*Some estimates and the number of cases in Yates are much higher than the total shown here.

Source: Leonard A. Jason, "An Illness That's Hard to Live with—or Define," *Wall Street Journal*, March 5, 2011. http://online.wsj.com.

- According to the CFIDS Association of America, **teenagers** are more likely than younger children to fit the diagnostic criteria for CFS established by the CDC.

What Causes Chronic Fatigue Syndrome?

❝The attempt to find one cause for all people with CFS is a fruitless exercise, just as the attempt to find one cause of depression, pneumonia, diabetes, or cancer is fruitless.❞

—Robert J. Hedaya, clinical professor of psychiatry at Georgetown University Hospital and founder of the National Center for Whole Psychiatry.

❝For a long time, the majority of studies focused on physical causes of CFS. More recent studies have started addressing mental-emotional factors as well. . . . In general, CFS is said to be a multifactorial disease, one in which many factors integrate together to create the symptoms.❞

—Daivati Bharadvaj, a naturopathic (natural medicine) physician from Portland, Oregon, and author of *Natural Treatments for Chronic Fatigue Syndrome*.

Scientists have studied CFS for decades, but the cause of this perplexing illness remains unknown. Many suspect that it has viral origins, as studies of CFS patients have shown that most have been infected with one or more viruses. Also, the characteristics of CFS closely resemble those of viral illnesses such as influenza, as the University of Maryland Medical Center explains: "In up to 80% of cases, chronic fatigue syndrome starts suddenly with a flu-like condition."[39] Just as the flu is highly contagious, some researchers suspect that the same might also be true of CFS, although this has never been proved. The group writes: "There is no evidence that CFS is spread through casual contact, such as shaking hands or coughing, or by intimate sexual contact."[40] Yet even without solid evidence, the possible contagion factor is still of interest to scientists. All reported outbreaks have begun with a few people getting sick, followed by a spread of the illness to others in the same workplace, school, or community. How can this be explained, many wonder, if CFS is not a contagious illness?

An example of how CFS spread throughout a community is the 1984 epidemic in Incline Village, Nevada, which was the subject of one of the largest CFS studies ever done. A January 1992 article published in *Annals of Internal Medicine* described several groups of patients who became ill within several months of each other, including 11 people who worked together at a casino, as well as students and teachers from three different high schools. The authors explained in the article

> " An example of how CFS spread throughout a community is the 1984 epidemic in Incline Village, Nevada, which was the subject of one of the largest CFS studies ever done. "

that many people who were stricken with the illness had family members who also got sick: "The spouses or sexual contacts of six patients were similarly afflicted, and there were at least eight instances in which one parent and one child both had the illness."[41] Yet as much as such factors might suggest that CFS can be transmitted from one person to another, this remains a possibility rather than a certainty.

The Infection Connection

One of the diagnostic terms that is often used in place of *chronic fatigue syndrome* is *chronic fatigue and immune dysfunction syndrome*, with the implication being that the illness results from an immune system that is not working properly. Studies have found many irregularities in the immune systems of people who suffer from CFS, which makes them vulnerable to infections that their bodies would normally be able to fight off. Robert H. Shmerling, clinical chief in the Rheumatology Division at Beth Israel Deaconess Medical Center in Boston, writes: "Infection has long been considered a possible cause of CFS. This hasn't been proven, but it's understandable that an infection—one that the immune system cannot completely eliminate—would be the prime suspect." Yet even without proof that CFS is caused by infectious agents, says Shmerling, "that does not rule out the possibility that a chronic infection (or the "fallout" from an infection) is to blame."[42]

Researchers from the Stanford School of Medicine have aggressively pursued studies to determine whether CFS results from an infection, and they have arrived at two possible theories. One is that the illness could be triggered by the persistent activity of a pathogen such as a bacterium or virus, and the second theory is that CFS may develop due to the body's immune response to the pathogen, rather than by the pathogen itself. The group writes: "Clinical, scientific and epidemiological [population-based] observations made by several research groups, including our own, have led to the development of these hypotheses. From an epidemiological perspective, it has been known for many years that the onset of CFS is often acute and preceded by a viral or infection-like illness."[43]

> " One of the diagnostic terms that is often used in place of *chronic fatigue syndrome* is *chronic fatigue and immune dysfunction syndrome*, with the implication being that the illness results from an immune system that is not working properly. "

According to the Stanford group, many infectious pathogens associated with CFS can affect the central nervous system, which is significant because cognitive impairment (poor mental function) is a common feature of the illness. The group writes: "It is possible that a chronic infection or inflammation in the brain may result in diminished cognitive capacity in these patients."[44] The group adds that along with cognitive difficulties, many CFS patients have gastrointestinal problems, with as many as 92 percent suffering from irritable bowel syndrome. Research by infectious disease specialist John Chia suggests that this could be due to infection by enteroviruses, which are viruses that typically affect the gastrointestinal tract. In one study, Chia's team found enterovirus protein in 82 percent of stomach biopsy samples from CFS patients and also in biopsy specimens that were taken years later. These sorts of studies strengthen the theory that pathogens may play a role in the development of CFS.

Immunity Under Attack

The possibility that CFS could result from an immune system gone awry has intrigued scientists for years. Recent studies have focused on a virus called HHV-6, because it is known to be connected to immune dysfunction. HHV-6, which is part of the herpes virus family, is extremely common. According to Shmerling, 95 percent of adults have been infected with it at some point during their childhood. But because the virus can remain dormant in the body for many years, it could flare up later in life. So, if someone infected with HHV-6 sustains immune system damage, he or she might be more susceptible to being stricken with CFS. Says Shmerling, "It should not be surprising that this virus would be a focus of study for CFS researchers."[45]

One way that HHV-6 disrupts the immune system is by causing alterations in cytokines. These are chemical messengers that send signals to immune cells (white blood cells), directing them to travel to infection sites and destroy foreign invaders. The right balance of cytokines is essential for proper immune system function: too few and the body's ability to fight off infection and disease is weakened, while too many sends the immune system into overdrive—and that can be dangerous. Cytokines spring into action, signaling the immune system to start pumping out white blood cells in order to fend off what has been mistaken for an attack by foreign invaders. In an ironic turn of events, the white blood cells become the body's worst enemy. They flood the bloodstream and launch an attack against the immune system itself, causing problems that range from inflammation to organ and tissue damage.

Viral Companions?

One of the viruses that repeatedly shows up in tests of people with CFS is the Epstein-Barr virus (EBV), which is another of the herpes viruses. The presence of EBV in someone's blood is not at all unusual, as it is one of the most common viruses that exist. According to the CDC, most people become infected with EBV at some point during their lives:

> In the United States, as many as 95% of adults between 35 and 40 years of age have been infected. Infants become susceptible to EBV as soon as maternal antibody protection (present at birth) disappears. Many children become infected with EBV, and these infections usually cause no symptoms or are indistinguishable from the other mild, brief illnesses of childhood.[46]

The CDC adds that when infection with EBV occurs during adolescence or young adulthood, it causes mononucleosis up to 50 percent of the time. This is significant in terms of CFS because many people who have mono go on to develop CFS.

Studies have shown that the likelihood of CFS following mono is highest among young people, as the authors of a July 2009 article in *Pediatrics* write: "Acute, mononucleosis-like illnesses preceding chronic fatigue have been documented for approximately three fourths of adolescents with CFS, with nearly one half exhibiting active mononucleosis infection at symptom onset."[47] The article discussed a study that examined the connection between mono and CFS in youth. A team of researchers from Chicago followed the progress of 301 adolescents who had been diagnosed with mono. After 6 months the team identified 53 youths who had not yet recovered, and tests showed that 39 of them (13 percent of total study participants) had developed CFS. At the conclusion of the study, the researchers determined that rates of CFS among adolescents who had previously had mono were at least 20 times higher than rates found in the general adolescent population.

> " One of the viruses that repeatedly shows up in tests of people with CFS is the Epstein-Barr virus (EBV), which is another of the herpes viruses. "

Retrovirus Feud

Of all the discoveries related to potential causes of CFS, none has generated as much excitement—and controversy—as studies that involve the retrovirus xenotropic murine leukemia virus–related virus (XMRV). In October 2009 virologist Judy A. Mikovits and her colleagues made an announcement about a groundbreaking study in the field of CFS research. In a paper published in the journal *Science*, the team described the study, which involved examining CFS clusters in Nevada, Florida, and South Carolina. Blood samples were taken from 101 CFS patients, as well as 218 healthy people from a control group. When the samples were analyzed, the team found that XMRV was in the blood of 67 percent of patients with CFS, compared with less than 4 percent of the other group—meaning there was a strong likelihood that XMRV was closely connected to CFS.

These findings gave hope to CFS patients, who were elated to learn that a cause might have been found at long last. Anne Ursu, a writer from Cleveland, Ohio, who has suffered with CFS, told a reporter from the *New York Times*: "I just feel like the whole future has changed for us."[48] Many scientists were optimistic about the study, but they also warned that further research was needed before a link with XMRV could be confirmed. And more studies did follow—but rather than confirm the findings, one study after another found no link with the retrovirus.

> " Of all the discoveries related to potential causes of CFS, none has generated as much excitement—and controversy—as studies that involve the retrovirus xenotropic murine leukemia virus–related virus (XMRV). "

Articles began appearing in *Science* and other professional journals denouncing the findings reported by Mikovits and her team, saying that the research was deeply flawed. One December 2010 press release announcing a study by researchers from University College London and Oxford University bluntly stated: "Chronic Fatigue Syndrome Is Not Caused by XMRV."[49] A study led by Jay Levy, a University of California retrovirologist who was one of the first to isolate HIV, failed to find XMRV in 61 patients with confirmed diagnosis of CFS—including 43 who were notified by the Mikovits group that they tested positive for the virus. By June 2011 at least 10 published studies reported a failure to detect XMRV in CFS patients, and the original study had been scientifically discredited.

Based on what was perceived as overwhelming evidence, the editors of *Science* asked Mikovits and her colleagues to voluntarily retract their paper. But being steadfastly convinced that their results were valid, the team refused and sharply criticized those who had challenged them. Jonathan Stoye, a retrovirologist from the United Kingdom, initially supported the original study and published his endorsement. But after being part of a research team that found no trace of XMRV in blood samples of over 500 study participants, Stoye became convinced that the Mikovits team's finding was flawed. He refers to their "endless succession" of criticisms about researchers who did not arrive at the same conclusion. "This isn't a conspiracy against them," he says. "Tens of labs have tried to reproduce their findings without success. There are some very smart people in this, and they would not have got this wrong. It's an insult to us all."[50]

Even with the radically different findings, however, the possible association of the XMRV retrovirus with CFS has by no means been discarded. Two studies organized by the National Institutes of Health are evaluating blood samples from CFS patients and healthy members of a control group to determine whether XMRV indeed has links to the illness, and the Mikovits team is participating in the research. In a June 2011 column published in *Science*, editor in chief Bruce Alberts expressed his concern about the original research but also spoke of optimism: "*Science* eagerly awaits the outcome of these further studies and will take appropriate action when their results are known."[51]

Many Questions, Few Answers

Since scientists first became aware of CFS, they have searched for answers about what might cause it. Research has revealed a number of possible contributors, including a dysfunctional immune system, infections, viruses, and retroviruses. Although none of these theories has proved to be conclusive, each study furthers scientific knowledge and understanding. Perhaps this pursuit will someday yield results, and CFS sufferers will no longer have to hear "I'm sorry but no one knows" when they ask why they are so sick.

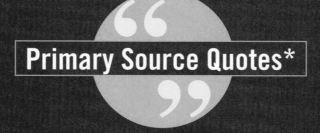

What Causes Chronic Fatigue Syndrome?

> **66** **The recent identification of xenotropic murine leukemia virus–related virus (XMRV) in the blood of patients with chronic fatigue syndrome (CFS) establishes that a retrovirus may play a role in the pathology in this disease.99**

—Vincent Lombardi and Judy A. Mikovits et al., "Xenotropic Murine Leukemia Virus–Related Virus–Associated Chronic Fatigue Syndrome Reveals a Distinct Inflammatory Signature," *In Vivo*, May 2011. http://merutt.files.wordpress.com.

Lombardi and Mikovits are researchers with the Whittemore Peterson Institute for Neuro-Immune Disease in Reno, Nevada.

> **66** **Despite [researcher Judy] Mikovits' claims, the evidence is very clear that she is wrong. Study after study has found no trace of the virus in CFS patients.99**

—Steven Salzberg, "Chronic Fatigue Syndrome: Virus Hypothesis Collapses Further," *Fighting Pseudoscience* (blog), *Forbes*, June 2, 2011. http://blogs.forbes.com.

Salzberg is a professor of medicine and biostatistics at the Johns Hopkins University's Institute of Genetic Medicine.

Bracketed quotes indicate conflicting positions.

* Editor's Note: While the definition of a primary source can be narrowly or broadly defined, for the purposes of Compact Research, a primary source consists of: 1) results of original research presented by an organization or researcher; 2) eyewitness accounts of events, personal experience, or work experience; 3) first-person editorials offering pundits' opinions; 4) government officials presenting political plans and/or policies; 5) representatives of organizations presenting testimony or policy.

"Whatever causes CFS . . . remains a mystery, and a troubling concern for patients who suffer from symptoms, which are often inconsistent with what laboratory tests and examinations can actually find."

—Stanford School of Medicine, "Hope for Chronic Fatigue Syndrome," Spring 2011. http://medicine.stanford.edu.

The Stanford School of Medicine specializes in patient care, biomedical research, professional education, and training.

"The XMRV virus study clearly documents that CFS is a real and physical illness, again proving that those who abuse patients by implying that the disease is all in their mind are being cruel and unscientific nitwits."

—Jacob Teitelbaum, "Got CFS? Dr. Oz Tackles the XMRV Virus," *The Dr. Oz Show*, December 4, 2009. www.doctoroz.com.

Teitelbaum, who recovered from CFS in 1975, is now medical director of the Fibromyalgia and Fatigue Centers.

"We have numerous theories about the possible causes of CFS, and yet not a single one has been fully endorsed by medical science as the principal cause of this elusive and life-altering syndrome."

—Jonathan E. Prousky, *The Vitamin Cure: For Chronic Fatigue Syndrome*. Laguna Beach, CA: Basic Health, 2010.

Prousky is a neuropathic practitioner at the Canadian College of Naturopathic Medicine in Toronto.

"All of us with C.F.S. have long felt that a virus is involved. The symptoms are so viral. You get fevers and chills and aching, a very sore throat, huge lymph nodes, and all the things you would get with flu, times ten, and they never go away."

—Laura Hillenbrand, "Back Issues: Laura Hillenbrand," *New Yorker*, October 15, 2009. www.newyorker.com.

Hillenbrand, the author of the books *Seabiscuit* and *Unbroken*, has suffered from severe CFS since she was 19 years old.

❝Despite extensive research to identify an infectious cause, there is no conclusive evidence that CFS is an infectious illness.❞

—Robert H. Shmerling, "Chronic Fatigue Syndrome: Names and Claims," Aetna InteliHealth, May 26, 2009. www.intelihealth.com.

Shmerling is clinical chief in the Rheumatology Division at Boston's Beth Israel Deaconess Medical Center.

❝There is no known cause for CFS, and most terrifying from where I sit, no cure.❞

—John Falk, "Chronic Fatigue Syndrome and Psychotherapy," *Huffington Post*, March 1, 2011. www.huffingtonpost.com.

Falk is a journalist and author who suffered from CFS for more than three years before he told anyone about his illness.

❝Studies of CFS have documented abnormalities in the immune, endocrine, autonomic nervous and central nervous systems.❞

—CFIDS Association of America, "Fiscal Year 2011 Appropriations Requests: Department of Defense," 2010. www.cfids.org.

The CFIDS Association of America is a charitable organization dedicated to ending the pain, suffering, and disability caused by CFS.

❝Studies suggest that CFS may be caused by inflammation along the nervous system, and that this inflammation may be some sort of immune response or process.❞

—National Institutes of Health, "Chronic Fatigue Syndrome," February 7, 2010. www.nlm.nih.gov.

The National Institutes of Health is the leading medical research agency in the United States.

❝When consistent biological findings do not emerge, investigators might inappropriately conclude that CFS is only a psychiatric problem.❞

—Leonard A. Jason, "An Illness That's Hard to Live with—or Define," *Wall Street Journal*, March 5, 2011. http://online.wsj.com.

Jason, a psychology professor and director of the Center for Community Research at DePaul University, was diagnosed with CFS in 1990.

What Causes Chronic Fatigue Syndrome?

- The CFIDS Association of America states that from **10 to 15 percent** of CFS patients have a family member who also has the illness, which suggests that genetics may play a role.

- According to the University of Maryland Medical Center, in patients with CFS, researchers have discovered **88 different genes** that are related to blood disease, immune system function, and infection.

- A study published in 2009 by researchers from Chicago found that **9 to 12 percent** of adults develop CFS after having mononucleosis.

- The CDC says that infection by EBV, Ross River virus, and *Coxiella burnetii* virus have all been shown to lead to a condition that meets the criteria for CFS in approximately **12 percent** of cases.

- According to the University of Maryland Medical Center, some studies have found that most CFS patients have **allergies** to certain foods, pollen, or metals such as mercury or nickel, which could trigger immune system abnormalities.

- A study published in July 2009 by researchers from Chicago found that rates of CFS among adolescents who had mononucleosis were at least **20 times higher** than rates found in the general adolescent population.

Many Possible Causes

Scientists do not know what causes chronic fatigue syndrome, although they have offered numerous theories. Most suspect a combination of factors contribute to chronic fatigue syndrome.

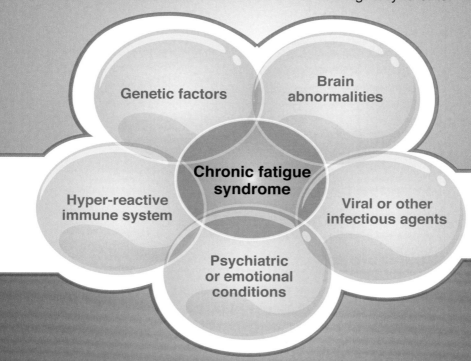

Genetic factors

Brain abnormalities

Chronic fatigue syndrome

Hyper-reactive immune system

Viral or other infectious agents

Psychiatric or emotional conditions

Source: University of Maryland Medical Center, "Chronic Fatigue Syndrome—Causes," January 13, 2009. www.umm.edu.

- An article published in 2009 by researchers from Israel states that the **human parvovirus B19** (which attacks the bones and red blood cells) has reportedly been associated with CFS more than any other virus.

- According to the CDC, several studies have shown that people with CFS have fewer of the white blood cells known as **natural killer cells** in their bodies than do healthy individuals.

The Link Between CFS and Mononucleosis

Studies have shown that teenagers who suffer from mononucleosis are more likely to develop chronic fatigue syndrome than those who have not had mono. This was the focus of a study published in the journal *Pediatrics* in July 2009. The study, which involved 301 adolescents aged 12 to 18, looked at the number who were diagnosed with CFS 6 months after having mono compared with the usual rate of CFS among adolescents.

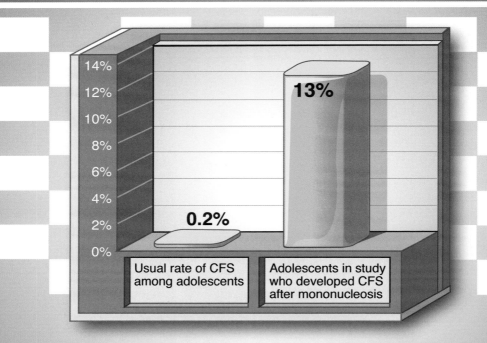

Source: Ben Z. Katz et al., "Chronic Fatigue Syndrome After Infectious Mononucleosis in Adolescents," *Pediatrics*, July 2009. http://pediatrics.aappublications.org.

- In a 2010 study published in the journal *Psychotherapy and Psychosomatics*, **28 percent** of participants with CFS had at least one personality disorder, with the most common being obsessive-compulsive disorder.

- According to the HHV-6 Foundation, the **herpes virus HHV-6** has been linked to several illnesses, including multiple sclerosis, epilepsy, and CFS.

A Possible Viral Link

Scientists have long suspected that CFS may be caused by one or more viruses, although a specific connection has not been found. In a study published in August 2010 by researchers from the Center for Biologics Evaluation and Research, National Institutes of Health Clinical Center, and Harvard Medical School, the majority of CFS patients tested positive for retroviruses called murine leukemia viruses (MLV). This finding does not prove that MLV causes CFS, but it is a potential connection that researchers intend to pursue. This graph illustrates the presence of the viruses in CFS patients compared with those in the healthy control group.

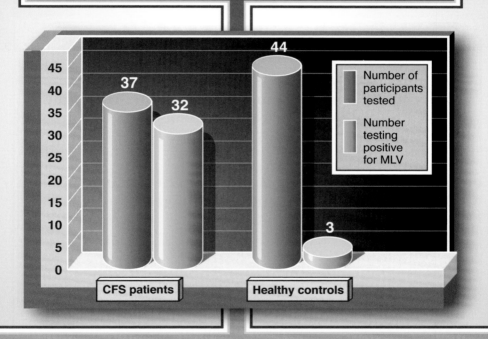

Source: US Food and Drug Administration, "Study: Presence of Murine Leukemia Virus Related Gene Sequences Found in CFS Patients," August 23, 2010. www.fda.gov.

- A 2009 study by researchers from the CDC and Emory University School of Medicine found that **childhood trauma** (sexual abuse and emotional maltreatment) was associated with a six-fold increased risk for CFS.

What Are the Effects of Chronic Fatigue Syndrome?

> **For most patients, CFS is a one-way ticket to hell. The affliction is acute and mostly incurable. Horrifically, it takes away even life's littlest pleasures.**
>
> —Llewellyn King, a veteran journalist and executive producer of the PBS news and public affairs program *White House Chronicle*.

> **For the sufferer CFS means a total health breakdown, like a plane that inexplicably begins tearing itself apart mid-flight.**
>
> —John Falk, a journalist and author who suffered from CFS for more than three years before he told anyone about his illness.

At the age of 18, Ben Di Pasquale thought life was pretty good. He was active in sports, did well in school, and enjoyed hanging out with his friends. In 2006 he graduated from Churchville Chili High School in Chili, New York, and that fall he started college—but after just one semester, Di Pasquale's whole world came crashing down. He was suddenly plagued by exhaustion like he had never known before, and even the simplest activity seemed overwhelming. He tried to get together with his friends but was too sick to be away from home for even an hour. "I would come home and crash," he says, "and I'd be in bed for the next couple of days just aching and exhausted."[52] None of the doctors Di Pasquale saw had any idea what was wrong with him. He was told to take more vitamins and get more exercise, but when he followed that advice he only got worse. Finally, Dr. David Bell diagnosed him with CFS.

Today Di Pasquale is 23 years old and almost totally bedridden. At 6 feet 2 inches tall (188 cm), he is down to a skeletal 118 pounds (53.5 kg). He is dependent on others to wash his hair and cut up his food when he eats, and when he is able to walk even a few steps—which is on a good day—he must lean on a cane. During 2010 Di Pasquale left his house on only 2 occasions, and was in a wheelchair both times. On Facebook he reads about all the fun things his friends are doing and wishes so badly that he could be with them. But he has no idea whether he will ever get better and have a normal life again. "This is my reality," he says, "and it might be too much for some people to take."[53]

Physical Agony

One of the most debilitating problems for many who suffer from CFS is having to cope with chronic pain. For some it is a dull ache in certain areas such as the face and behind the eyes, while others feel pain throughout the entire body. Molly Billings falls into the latter category. Her head hurts constantly, she aches all over, and sometimes her joints feel "like the marrow has worn away and my bones are scraping against each other." Billings's experience has taught her that the pain associated with CFS is a unique kind of pain, as she writes: "When you prick yourself with a pin, or accidentally cut yourself, you feel a very specific kind of pain. You can point to the place on your body where it hurts and can tell exactly what you are feeling. That is not the case with CFS." Billings describes her own pain as being "like a constant white noise. I always feel a sensation of discomfort. You feel it in every movement and every cell. There is no relief or break."[54]

> " One of the most debilitating problems for many who suffer from CFS is having to cope with chronic pain. "

Lindsey Dunlap is familiar with the concept of never-ending pain because it describes her life. Now 24 years old, Dunlap has suffered from CFS since she was a teenager about to start her senior year in high school. On the first day of classes, she felt faint, nauseous, dizzy, and overwhelmingly exhausted. "That first day just so happened to be the last day I was ever able to attend any classes my entire senior year," she says. Today Dunlap is in constant pain "every hour of every day." She explains:

> Something as simple as stretching to reach high in a cupboard can cause me severe muscle pain for days. I'm so sensitive that my bed has to have piles of mattress toppers because even my very soft bed feels like I am trying to sleep on a slab of concrete. I joke that the princess from the fairy tale "The Princess and the Pea" must have had Chronic Fatigue Syndrome because I too could not get a decent night of sleep sleeping on top of something as miniscule as a pea.[55]

The Heartache of Rejection

As if the physical problems of CFS were not enough to bear, many sufferers are also forced to cope with disbelief and even scorn from those who do not think the illness is real. This is distressing for those who suffer from it, which was the reason John Falk kept his illness to himself for more than three years. Falk is a journalist from New York who has traveled all over the world to cover stories for major publications such as *National Geographic*. He says that the reaction people typically have toward someone with CFS can be as difficult as the illness itself. "When you have CFS," he says, "one of the greatest battles you fight are the ignorant smirks and expressed disbelief of those who think it's all in your head; that is, those that don't live with you and live the truth of CFS everyday. Negativity and doubt amount to an energy drain you can ill afford. It's the reason I have refused up until now to identify myself as a person with CFS."[56]

Falk has found that negative attitudes about CFS are also shared by many medical professionals. He has seen four different therapists in an effort to come to terms with his frustrations over how the illness has affected his life, but all he has gained from the experience is added frustration. He writes: "I have found each time a good-natured, well-intended professional who—when I tell them my textbook symptoms of CFS—only shake their heads and say, I never heard of that. It must be awful. Thereafter I spend my money and more importantly my precious energy stores educating them on CFS while they in turn struggle to fit me into a paradigm of psychological dysfunction."[57]

Toni Bernhard can relate to Falk's experience. Once a successful university law professor, Bernhard has been debilitated by CFS since 2001, when she failed to recover from what seemed to be an acute viral infection. "It has left me mostly house-bound, often bed-bound," she says. "In effect, I've had the flu without the fever for almost ten years: the aches and pains, the dazed sick feeling, the low grade headache, the severe fatigue."[58] Yet as sick as she is, Bernhard repeatedly encounters physicians who have either not heard of CFS or scoff at it, believing it to be a product of a patient's imagination. When doctors ask about her health, she feels like she has been put in a "no-win position" as she explains: "If I say, 'I have Chronic Fatigue Syndrome,' I'm likely to be discredited as a witness to my own condition. I've had doctors tell me there's no such thing as Chronic Fatigue Syndrome. One doctor said: 'Just drink some coffee.'"[59]

> **As if the physical problems of CFS were not enough to bear, many sufferers are also forced to cope with disbelief and even scorn from those who do not think the illness is real.**

Bernhard recalls one visit to a doctor's office for a condition unrelated to CFS. She filled out a medical form and checked "no" to a question about whether she was in good health, and then provided the explanation: "Contracted a serious viral infection in 2001 and never recovered." In the examination room, the doctor was reviewing Bernhard's form and asked about the viral illness. She writes:

> Without using the phrase Chronic Fatigue Syndrome, I succinctly explained the different theories regarding the cause of my continued illness. He listened and then said: "What's the diagnosis?" I was cornered. "Chronic Fatigue Syndrome," I said. I watched him disengage from me. He swiveled on his stool, put his note pad down, turned back to me as if we'd just met and said: "What have you come to see me about today?"[60]

Careers Lost

According to the CDC, chronic fatigue syndrome can be just as disabling as diseases such as multiple sclerosis, rheumatoid arthritis, lupus, heart disease, and late-stage kidney disease. Many who suffer from the illness make every attempt to go on with their lives and careers but often find that to be impossible. This was the case with Laurel Bertrand. Three weeks after she was diagnosed with CFS, her condition had not improved much, but she was determined to go back to work because her temperature had dropped below 100°F (38°C). Instead of feeling better, though, her condition worsened. "Clearly, it was too soon." she says. "Within a month, my 104 fever was back full blown, and I was out of work for another 3 weeks."[61]

For the next few years, Bertrand continued to push herself hard, somehow managing to hold on to her full-time job. "I was running my body to the ground," she says, "and though I knew this, I did it anyway. I was of the mind-set that I could push through anything, and that with enough perseverance, I would eventually overcome. Not so." After years of pushing her body beyond its capacity, Bertrand suffered such a severe crash that she ended up having to quit her job. More difficulties lay ahead. She writes: "Not long after that, I had a crash that left me bedridden and unable to speak above a whisper. That was 9 years ago. I have spent what was supposed to be the most vital years of my life sick, barely able to speak and confined to my bedroom."[62]

> **Many who suffer from the illness make every attempt to go on with their lives and careers but often find that to be impossible.**

Samuel Salomaa also knows what it is like to be forced out of a career because of CFS. Before he got sick, he had worked at American Honda Motor Company in Southern California for more than 20 years. His coworkers and supervisors knew him as both intelligent and hardworking; he was also physically active, often walking or jogging to work. Then in 2003 Salomaa came down with what appeared to be the flu and stayed home for three days. When he returned to work, it was as though he had become a different person. Even the smallest tasks left him completely exhausted, and it was obvious to others that he was not thinking clearly. After seeing several doctors, Salomaa was diagnosed with CFS and was told that he had one of the worst cases they had ever seen. Because he was so sick, he could not continue working and had no choice but to quit his job.

When Kids Are Hurting

Even though young people suffer from CFS, the illness is much more common among adults. Because of that, few studies have focused on children and adolescents. The University of Maryland Medical Center writes: "Although children with symptoms of chronic fatigue have not been as rigorously studied as adults, limited evidence suggests that CFS can be significantly disabling in young people. Studies report that adolescents who meet the criteria for CFS also have greater anxiety, depression, and school absenteeism than their peers."[63]

One study that did focus on adolescents was published in the April 18, 2011, issue of *Pediatrics.* Researchers from the Netherlands conducted a comprehensive survey of physicians and found that among teenagers diagnosed with CFS, more than 90 percent had missed considerable time at school over a period of six months. Based on their findings, the team concluded that the illness can be extremely disabling in young people. British physician Katharine Rimes shares her thoughts:

> **Even though young people suffer from CFS, the illness is much more common among adults. Because of that, few studies have focused on children and adolescents.**

> Missing substantial amounts of school can potentially have profound effects on their educational, social and emotional development. It also has a potentially serious impact on the family. If the child is off school, one parent . . . usually has to stay at home to care for them, and often give up their job altogether. This can obviously have adverse financial and psychological effects.[64]

Fighting for Survival

CFS can tear people's lives apart. It results in crushing fatigue and unbearable pain and can rob people of their jobs, their relationships, their self-esteem—and life as they once knew it. Yet in spite of how devastating CFS can be, and as hard as they must struggle, some refuse to let go of their dreams. Bertrand writes: "I love to travel. I love to learn. I love to draw and read and spend time with friends and family. I love photography and the outdoors. I love to dance. It's not that I no longer want to do these things. It's that I can't."[65]

What Are the Effects of Chronic Fatigue Syndrome?

66 The experience of chronic fatigue syndrome varies from person to person. For many people, however, the symptoms are more bothersome early in the course of the illness and then gradually decrease. 99

—Mayo Clinic, "Chronic Fatigue Syndrome," June 19, 2009. www.mayoclinic.com.

The Mayo Clinic is a world-renowned medical facility headquartered in Rochester, Minnesota.

66 When you have chronic fatigue syndrome, besides being bone-tired, you may experience headaches, muscle and joint pain, and insomnia and other symptoms. 99

—Chrystle Fiedler, *The Complete Idiot's Guide to Natural Remedies*. New York: Penguin, 2009.

Fiedler is a writer who specializes in health-related topics and natural remedies.

* Editor's Note: While the definition of a primary source can be narrowly or broadly defined, for the purposes of Compact Research, a primary source consists of: 1) results of original research presented by an organization or researcher; 2) eyewitness accounts of events, personal experience, or work experience; 3) first-person editorials offering pundits' opinions; 4) government officials presenting political plans and/or policies; 5) representatives of organizations presenting testimony or policy.

Primary Source Quotes

❝We are the walking dead. Some of us are so close to death that it's like lying in a grave that has already been dug, desperately holding onto one strand of grass.❞

—Lori Chapo-Kroger, testimony before the US Department of Health and Human Services Chronic Fatigue Syndrome Advisory Committee, May 11, 2011. www.hhs.gov.

Chapo-Kroger is a registered nurse who founded CFS Solutions of West Michigan.

❝A person with CFS may have muscle pain, trouble focusing, or insomnia (not being able to sleep). The extreme tiredness may come and go. In some cases the extreme tiredness never goes away.❞

—National Women's Health Information Center, "Chronic Fatigue Syndrome," September 22, 2009. www.womenshealth.gov.

The National Women's Health Information Center is dedicated to improving the health and well-being of all women and girls in the United States.

❝This disease leaves people bedridden. I've gone through phases where I couldn't roll over in bed. I couldn't speak. To have it called 'fatigue' is a gross misnomer.❞

—Laura Hillenbrand, interviewed by Tara Parker-Pope, "An Author Escapes from Chronic Fatigue Syndrome," *Well* (blog), *New York Times*, February 4, 2011. http://well.blogs.nytimes.com.

Hillenbrand, the author of the books *Seabiscuit* and *Unbroken*, has suffered from severe CFS since she was 19 years old.

❝Living with ME/CFS is a constant struggle. We can't escape it even for a day because we can't escape our bodies and our limitations. It is always there and we worry that it will always BE there, and there's nothing we can do about it.❞

—Sue Jackson, "My Testimony for CFSAC," *Learning to Live with CFS* (blog), April 19, 2011. http://livewithcfs.blogspot.com.

Jackson has had CFS for 10 years and has two teenage sons who also suffer from the illness.

"My H.I.V. patients for the most part are hale and hearty thanks to three decades of intense and excellent research and billions of dollars invested. Many of my C.F.S. patients, on the other hand, are terribly ill and unable to work or participate in the care of their families."

—Nancy G. Klimas, "Readers Ask: A Virus Linked to Chronic Fatigue Syndrome," *Consults* (blog), *New York Times*, October 15, 2009. http://consults.blogs.nytimes.com.

Klimas is director of the Department of Immunology of the University of Miami School of Medicine and a member of the board of the International Association for Chronic Fatigue Syndrome.

"My bones are so osteoporotic that every cough and sneeze could cause a fracture. How can I live the life I have dreamed of; swimming, sailing, running, cycling. The kind of life I had before it was taken away from me at the age of 14."

—Lynn Gilderdale, "Lynn Gilderdale's Moving Account of Why She Decided to End Her Life," *Sunday Times* (London), January 26, 2010. www.timesonline.co.uk.

Gilderdale committed suicide after suffering from CFS for more than 15 years.

"This disabling fatigue is accompanied by: unrestorative sleep, problems with concentration and short-term memory, joint and muscle pain, tender lymph nodes, sore throat and headache."

—CFIDS Association of America, "Fiscal Year 2011 Appropriations Requests: Department of Defense," 2010. www.cfids.org.

The CFIDS Association of America is a charitable organization dedicated to ending the pain, suffering, and disability caused by CFS.

What Are the Effects of Chronic Fatigue Syndrome?

- According to the CFIDS Association of America, population-based studies of CFS have found that at least **25 percent** of sufferers are either unemployed or receiving disability.

- A study published in May 2011 by researchers from the Netherlands found that **90 percent** of teens with CFS had significant school absences, defined by missing school at least **15 percent** of the time.

- According to the Stanford School of Medicine, studies have shown that up to **90 percent** of CFS patients suffer from gastrointestinal problems of varying severity.

- A 2009 report published in the Veterans' Law Review stated that thousands of veterans of the **Persian Gulf War** experienced symptoms consistent with CFS, including back pain, joint pain, sleep difficulties, headaches, and excessive fatigue.

- A study published in July 2009 by researchers from Chicago stated that CFS causes significant functional impairment and **educational disruption** among adolescents who suffer from the illness.

- According to the CFIDS Association of America, from **20 percent to 44 percent** of children with CFS must be homeschooled because they are too ill to attend classes.

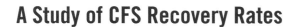

A Study of CFS Recovery Rates

One of the most well known outbreaks of chronic fatigue syndrome occurred between 1984 and 1987 in Lyndonville, New York. In the years since, the physician who treated the patients, David S. Bell, has followed their progress. This chart shows what he has discovered about their recovery as of 2011.

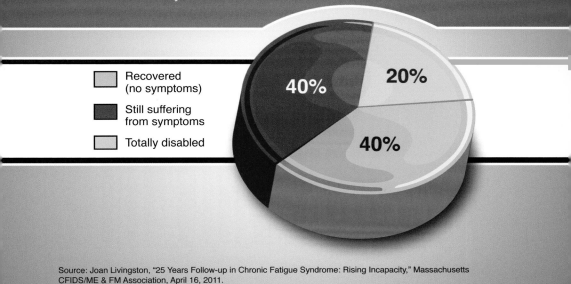

Recovered (no symptoms)

Still suffering from symptoms

Totally disabled

20%

40%

40%

Source: Joan Livingston, "25 Years Follow-up in Chronic Fatigue Syndrome: Rising Incapacity," Massachusetts CFIDS/ME & FM Association, April 16, 2011.

- The CDC states that annual medical costs for an individual suffering from CFS are about **$3,200**.

- According to the Stanford School of Medicine, studies have shown that **35 to 92 percent** of CFS patients suffer from irritable bowel syndrome.

- A study by researchers from Chicago found that participants with CFS were more likely to be receiving **disability income, be unemployed, or be working part-time** than healthy individuals in the control group.

How CFS Affects Quality of Life

To examine the effects of chronic fatigue syndrome on young people, researchers in the United Kingdom performed a study that involved 25 youth with CFS and 23 healthy youth between the ages of 10 and 18. Based on information compiled from questionnaires, the team determined that CFS significantly impaired a sufferer's quality of life compared with that of healthy young people, as well as those with diabetes or asthma.

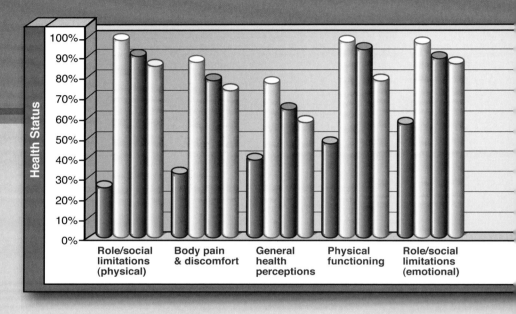

- According to the international advocacy organization Hummingbird Foundation for M.E., from **25 to 30 percent** of CFS sufferers are housebound, wheelchair bound, and/or bedridden.

- According to the CDC, productivity lost to the US economy because of CFS is from **$1 million to $4 million** annually.

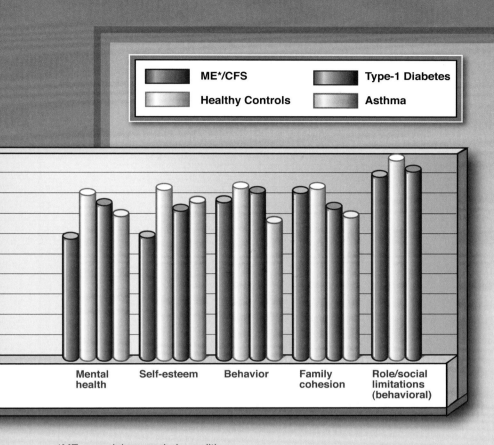

Legend: ME*/CFS, Healthy Controls, Type-1 Diabetes, Asthma

Categories: Mental health, Self-esteem, Behavior, Family cohesion, Role/social limitations (behavioral)

*ME = myalgic encephalomyelitis.

Note: Higher scores indicate better health status.

Source: ME Research, "The Quality of Life of Children with ME/CFS," *Breakthrough*, Spring 2010. www.mcresearch.org.uk.

- A 2010 study of CFS sufferers from Georgia found that the disease accounted for **$8,554** in annual lost household earnings.

- A study published in 2011 by researchers from Turkey found that the incidence of **pain, sleep disturbances, and social isolation** among CFS sufferers was more than double that of healthy participants.

CFS Leads to High Absenteeism from School

One of the most difficult problems for young people who suffer from CFS is that they often miss a lot of school, which not only affects their grades but also their social development. This was the focus of a study published in April 2011 by researchers from the Netherlands, who examined a group of Dutch adolescents aged 10 to 18 who suffered from CFS. The team found that the young people with CFS missed a considerable amount of school when compared with their healthy peers.

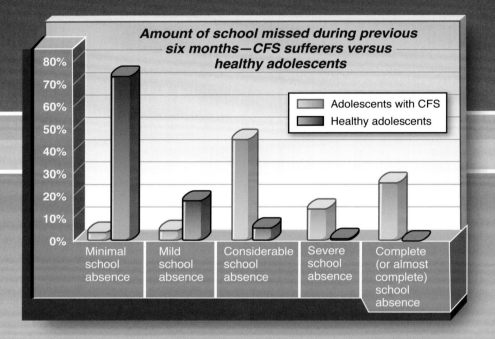

Amount of school missed during previous six months—CFS sufferers versus healthy adolescents

Legend:
- Adolescents with CFS
- Healthy adolescents

Categories: Minimal school absence, Mild school absence, Considerable school absence, Severe school absence, Complete (or almost complete) school absence

Source: Sane L. Nijhof et al., "Adolescent Chronic Fatigue Syndrome: Prevalence, Incidence, and Morbidity," *Pediatrics*, May 2011. http://pediatrics.aappublications.org.

Can People Overcome Chronic Fatigue Syndrome?

❝I am convinced that chronic fatigue syndrome . . . can be managed successfully. I believe that the medical profession will rise to the task of addressing this illness properly. I also feel that there will be treatments in the future that will completely reverse the symptoms.❞

—David S. Bell, a general medicine physician from Lyndonville, New York, who has treated a large number of patients with CFS.

❝Some patients never return to their pre-illness state. Most studies report that patients who are treated in an extensive rehabilitation program are more likely to recover completely than those patients who don't seek treatment.❞

—National Institutes of Health, the leading medical research agency in the United States.

It is impossible for health officials to know with any certainty how many people recover from CFS. A major reason is that only about 20 percent of CFS sufferers seek treatment, so most are never diagnosed. Other factors also come into play, as the University of Maryland Medical Center explains:

> Because the illness remains elusive and poorly defined, and there are few objective measures for recovery, experts

have found it difficult to determine the long-term course of the disease. Many patients are not covered by insurance or have difficulty finding good care, so available statistics may be incorrect. Bearing these factors in mind, some studies have reported that more than half of patients who complain of chronic fatigue are still fatigued at 2 years. Although a variety of studies have attempted to identify factors that predict a more chronic or severe course, no clear conclusions can be made.[66]

Challenges and Triumphs

People with CFS face innumerable difficulties, from having an illness that is often scoffed at to suffering from pain and crushing fatigue. One of their biggest challenges is that no treatment exists for the illness itself. Unlike many diseases for which antibiotics or other curative drugs can be prescribed, the same is not true for CFS. The CDC writes: "Managing chronic fatigue syndrome can be as complex as the illness itself. There is no cure, no prescription drugs have been developed specifically for CFS, and symptoms vary considerably over time."[67] The CDC adds that treatments are developed on an individual basis and are frequently revised based on how effective they may or may not be. Treatment often includes a combination of exercise therapy, medication to relieve symptoms, and counseling to help patients cope with the difficulties of their illness.

> **People with CFS face innumerable difficulties, from having an illness that is often scoffed at to suffering from pain and crushing fatigue. One of their biggest challenges is that no treatment exists for the illness itself.**

Robert Gonzalez, a man from California whose wife, Sandi, has CFS, calls it a "dastardly illness" from which she has not fully recovered. But through treatment—combined with her own fierce determination to get better—she has seen dramatic improvement, as he writes: "She still has bad days, but at the end of the day, she is doing worlds better now than she was just two years ago."[68] As with many CFS patients, Sandi saw a doctor who prescribed medications for the various symptoms of her illness. This made a considerable difference in her ability to sleep and her overall physical health, as well as her peace of mind. Also, she started to watch her diet and became more physically active, as Robert explains: "I don't know if this was a matter of willpower or a renewed sense of energy but activity actually helped her get more active which continued to help her improve."[69]

> **Many who suffer from CFS are offended at the very mention of mental or emotional issues, interpreting that to mean that they are not really sick and the illness is 'all in their heads.'**

According to Robert, a major change for his wife was forcing herself to develop a new outlook on life, separating what is important from what is not. "That may sound almost lame to have to say that," he says, "but one of the things that seemed to cause her a lot of stress was worry over the things that were going on at home, with the kids, with our money and with our family."[70] Once Sandi made a concerted effort to rid herself of the stress that was weighing her down, Robert says he could actually see her develop a new sense of peace. And a significant part of her progress was due to her faith, as he explains: "She prayed. A lot. . . . If you are a religious/spiritual person then prayer will be invaluable to you. It was to her, and she would attest to that fact."[71]

Even though Sandi still has a long way to go before she is completely recovered, her family has witnessed incredible progress. "While she has made tremendous strides in healing," says Robert, "she will admit that she still has bad days here and there. Still, she has plenty more good days than bad and she strives every day to make each day count."[72]

Treating Mind and Body

One of the most contentious aspects of CFS is whether its cause can be somewhat attributed to psychological factors. Many who suffer from CFS are offended at the very mention of mental or emotional issues, interpreting that to mean that they are not really sick and the illness is "all in their heads." And because CFS sufferers often encounter that sort of negativity—even among medical professionals—it is understandable that they would be wary of any treatment that focuses on the mind rather than the body. Michael Sharpe, a psychiatrist and professor at the University of Edinburgh in Scotland, explains: "If you have a condition that people decry and criticize you for, saying it's not really real, it's just psychological, then someone tells you, 'You need a psychological treatment,' it seems like rubbing it in, that people don't believe they're ill."[73]

Robert J. Hedaya, who is also a psychiatrist, agrees that the primary treatment for CFS should not be psychotherapy because CFS is primarily a physical illness. But based on what he calls the "whole psychiatry" understanding of CFS, people need to realize that the mind and body work together in development of CFS. A successful treatment program, says Hedaya, will take that into consideration. He writes:

> You might wonder, if this is not a psychological or psychiatric problem, why would a psychiatrist treat it? The answer is two-fold. First, I myself have had chronic fatigue syndrome and recovered, and second, it was through the process of treating myself that Whole Psychiatry was born. Of course, as a result of my own learning, it became apparent that the body and mind are not separate, and are one entity which must be evaluated and treated simultaneously for the best outcome.[74]

A Treatment Breakthrough?

The value of treating the mind as well as the body was revealed in a major research project led by Sharpe. One of the largest studies ever conducted in the treatment of CFS, it involved 641 CFS patients. The findings were published in the British medical journal the *Lancet* in February 2011. The purpose of the study was to evaluate what treatment or combination of treatments was most effective. The patients all received specialized medical care, including disease education and medication to treat symptoms, and were then randomly divided into four groups. One group received no treatment beyond medical care, while those in the other groups also participated in one of three additional treatments.

These treatments included adaptive pacing, graded exercise therapy, and cognitive behavioral therapy (CBT). Adaptive pacing involves helping patients acknowledge their physical limitations while gradually increasing activity levels within their limits. Graded exercise therapy is a form of physical therapy that gradually increases in intensity over time, gently pushing a person to exceed what was accomplished in previous sessions. CBT is a type of psychotherapy that helps patients understand their individual symptoms and beliefs and develop strategies to improve day-to-day functioning. John Falk writes: "CBT is intended to help the patient deal with the ugly reality that they will never get better, that they are forever changed, and that the old you is gone and the new 'CFS you' needs to be embraced."[75]

The study lasted for a year. At its conclusion, the researchers found that CBT and graded exercise therapy showed markedly better results for patients than medical care alone or medical care combined with adaptive pacing. The latter is favored by most CFS specialists, but Sharpe's research found

> " The [CFS treatment] study lasted for a year. At its conclusion, the researchers found that CBT and graded exercise therapy showed markedly better results for patients than medical care alone or medical care combined with adaptive pacing. "

that it did not reduce fatigue or improve patients' ability to climb steps, walk longer distances, or engage in typical daily activities. He offers his thoughts about the findings: "I hope the results of this trial will go some way to reassuring some of those people that if this treatment is done by skilled people in an appropriate way, it actually is safe and can stand a very good chance of benefiting them." Sharpe acknowledges, however, that not everyone will have a favorable impression of what the study revealed: "There will be some who will be straightforwardly pleased. But I think there will be those who are more concerned and suspicious about it."[76]

Sharpe was correct in predicting that his research would be met with negative reactions. One who expressed scorn for the findings was Kim McCleary, president of the CFIDS Association of America. She explains:

> " **Recovering from CFS has been possible for some— but remains only a dream for others.** "

"The issue[s] with cognitive behavior therapy and graded exercise therapy . . . have to do with the impression that if these things are effective then it must mean that the condition is all in my head. If you can make it better by changing my illness beliefs, what you're saying to me [is] that I don't have a real illness or a physical illness."[77]

Graded exercise therapy is of particular concern to McLeary and other CFS advocates. While it may work for some patients, opponents of the technique say it implies that CFS sufferers could get out of bed and do more if they wanted to badly enough. Also, if they push themselves too hard, this can cause a crash, which sends them back to bed in worse shape than they were before.

Writing as an Escape

Laura Hillenbrand is well known among avid readers because she is the author of the books *Seabiscuit* and *Unbroken*. What many people do not realize, though, is that Hillenbrand is so debilitated by CFS that she can rarely leave her home. She has never personally met any of the people she writes about; instead, she interviews them on the telephone, and even that is physically taxing. "I've been too weak to leave the house for two years," she says. "I only leave the house about once a month. I'm just not very strong. A lot of days I don't get down the stairs." For Hillenbrand, getting lost in her writing provides a way to focus on something other than the illness that has taken over her life. "Physically, I can't escape this illness, or even this house," she says, "but when I'm writing, I'm not here; I am in another place and time, in another body, living through someone else."[78]

Hillenbrand has suffered from CFS since she was 19 years old and a sophomore in college. Because she was so sick, she had to drop out of school and was bedridden for 2 years. Since that time her illness has gone in cycles, with times that she felt better and others when she had severe crashes. In 1991 Hillenbrand felt well enough to take a road trip—and it resulted in what she calls a "catastrophic" CFS crash. She went into shock "and went back down to the bottom to worse than ever. Then vertigo started, and ever since the room appears to be moving around me. I feel like I'm moving all the time."[79] Hillenbrand never fully recovered from that, and she had yet another relapse in 2007. And while no treatment has helped her, being able to get lost in her books does:

> While it's really hard to do, at the same time, I'm escaping my body, which I really want to do. I'm living someone else's life. I get very intensely into the story, into the interviews and the research. I'm experiencing things along with my subjects. I have a freedom I don't have in my physical life. Writing is a godsend to me that way. Without it I wouldn't have anything.[80]

"The Battle Goes On"

Recovering from CFS has been possible for some—but remains only a dream for others. It is a challenging illness to treat, with no drugs or therapies that have proved to work for all CFS patients. As difficult as it is, many people with CFS accept that life as they once knew it is over without having any idea whether the future will be better or worse. Laurel Bertrand shares her thoughts: "Most of all, I dream of the vibrant, glorious feeling of good health. And I strive for it every day. In the meantime, I watch through my bedroom window as time slips by. The battle goes on."[81]

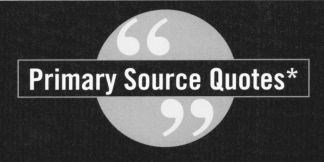

Can People Overcome Chronic Fatigue Syndrome?

> **Chronic fatigue syndrome is considered by most authorities to be a difficult-to-treat and elusive medical condition. However, there is much hope and optimism now because treatments are available to make a manageable chronic illness.**

—Jonathan E. Prousky, *The Vitamin Cure: For Chronic Fatigue Syndrome*. Laguna Beach, CA: Basic Health, 2010.

Prousky is the chief neuropathic medical officer at the Canadian College of Naturopathic Medicine in Toronto, Ontario.

> **The percentage of CFS patients who recover is unknown, but there is some evidence to indicate that the sooner a person is treated, the better the chance of improvement.**

—CDC, "Chronic Fatigue Syndrome," March 24, 2011. www.cdc.gov.

The CDC is dedicated to protecting health and promoting quality of life through the prevention and control of disease, injury, and disability.

* Editor's Note: While the definition of a primary source can be narrowly or broadly defined, for the purposes of Compact Research, a primary source consists of: 1) results of original research presented by an organization or researcher; 2) eyewitness accounts of events, personal experience, or work experience; 3) first-person editorials offering pundits' opinions; 4) government officials presenting political plans and/or policies; 5) representatives of organizations presenting testimony or policy.

> **Some people say their CFS symptoms get better with complementary or alternative treatments, such as massage, acupuncture, chiropractic care, yoga, stretching, or self-hypnosis.**

—National Women's Health Information Center, "Chronic Fatigue Syndrome: Frequently Asked Questions," September 22, 2009. www.womenshealth.gov.

The National Women's Health Information Center is dedicated to improving the health and well-being of all women and girls in the United States.

> **Above all, more needs to be done so that those of us stricken with the disease can have our lives back.**

—Laurel Bertrand, "My Story," *Dreams at Stake* (blog), May 25, 2009. http://dreamsatstake.blogspot.com.

Bertrand, who is in her late thirties, has suffered from severe CFS for 15 years.

> **I'm still fighting to get better and am not yet ready to surrender to a life where I spend 20 hours a day horizontal, lack the physical energy to sleep with my wife, and hold my new baby girl for more than a minute.**

—John Falk, "Chronic Fatigue Syndrome and Psychotherapy," *Huffington Post*, March 1, 2011. www.huffingtonpost.com.

Falk is a journalist and author who suffers from CFS.

> **I view chronic fatigue syndrome as a disorder of mind and body, not one or the other. Cognitive-behavior therapy does not cure chronic fatigue syndrome, but it can help—sometimes substantially.**

—Fred Friedberg, "Behavioral Treatments for Chronic Fatigue Syndrome," *Consults* (blog), *New York Times*, October 13, 2009. http://consults.blogs.nytimes.com.

Friedberg is a clinical psychologist and behavioral research scientist who is an assistant professor at New York's Stony Brook University Hospital.

"If you've got CFS you've got to fight for your health by pushing against your pain and exhaustion to get in better mental and physical shape."

—Charles Raison, "Mind-Body: Inside Chronic Fatigue," *The Chart* (blog), CNN, February 23, 2011. http://thechart.blogs.cnn.com.

Raison is an associate professor of psychiatry and behavioral sciences at Emory University and CNN's mental health expert.

"Preliminary studies indicate that for CFS, as with other chronic conditions, early detection, diagnosis and treatment ultimately yield better health outcomes."

—CFIDS Association of America, "Diagnosis: Do I Have CFS?," 2011. www.cfids.org.

The CFIDS Association of America is a charitable organization dedicated to ending the pain, suffering, and disability caused by CFS.

"For the past year and a half, I've been slowly, slowly improving, but it's been a long and difficult haul. I'm now well enough to get around my house fairly well on good days, and sometimes go out, but there are more bad days than good."

—Laura Hillenbrand, "Q&A with *Seabiscuit, Unbroken* Author Laura Hillenbrand," *Sports Illustrated*, December 15, 2010. http://sportsillustrated.cnn.com.

Hillenbrand, the author of the books *Seabiscuit* and *Unbroken*, has suffered from severe CFS since she was 19 years old.

"For patients who have been abandoned to quackish theories and harsh ideologies about their illness for 25 years, the dismantling of 'chronic fatigue syndrome' can't come soon enough."

—Hillary Johnson, "A Case of Chronic Denial," *New York Times*, October 20, 2009. www.nytimes.com.

Johnson is a journalist and the author of *Osler's Web: Inside the Labyrinth of the Chronic Fatigue Syndrome Epidemic*.

Facts and Illustrations

Can People Overcome Chronic Fatigue Syndrome?

- The CFIDS Association of America estimates that only about **20 percent** of CFS sufferers seek medical attention.

- The National Institutes of Health's 2012 estimated funding for CFS research is **$6 million**, compared with $3.2 billion for HIV/AIDS, $837 million for obesity, $461 million for alcoholism, $428 million for depression, and $253 million for arthritis.

- The CDC says there is some evidence showing that **the sooner a person is treated** for CFS, the **better the chance of improvement**.

- According to the CFIDS Association of America, long-term difficulties resulting from **cognitive disorders** may be more prevalent in children with CFS than adults because symptoms occur during a period of rapid intellectual development.

- In 2007 the Stanford School of Medicine announced a study in which 25 CFS patients were treated with a strong antiviral drug known as **Valcyte and 84 percent** improved dramatically.

- According to the University of Maryland Medical Center, **40 to 60 percent** of CFS patients suffer from memory impairments.

Treating Chronic Fatigue Syndrome

Because CFS affects people differently, no treatment exists that will work for everyone. The Centers for Disease Control and Prevention says that treatment programs are developed on an individual basis, with relief of symptoms being a primary treatment goal. This diagram shows some of the most common treatment options for CFS sufferers and what each is intended to accomplish.

Treatment Option	Intended Purpose
Professional counseling	Helps patients build effective coping skills; lessen anxiety, depression, grief, anger, and guilt often associated with chronic illness.
Cognitive behavioral therapy (CBT)	Helps patient overcome difficulties by changing dysfunctional thinking, behavior, and emotional responses.
Graded exercise therapy	Introduces physical activity very slowly, then gradually increases over time.
Alternative therapies	Deep breathing and muscle relaxation techniques, massage and movement therapies like yoga and tai chi.
Support groups	Can provide patient the ability to meet and share information with others who suffer from CFS.
Pharmacologic therapy	Directed toward relief of symptoms such as depression, sleep difficulties, cognitive problems, pain, and other specific problems.
Sleep hygiene	Can help CFS patients adopt good sleep habits.
Orthostatic instability therapy	Helps with symptoms such as dizziness, light-headedness, problems standing upright.

Source: Centers for Disease Control and Prevention, "Chronic Fatigue Syndrome: Treatment and Management Options," July 21, 2010. www.cdc.gov.

- In a 2010 study of 142 CFS patients by researcher A. Martin Lerner and his colleagues, **26 percent** of those who were given long-term antiviral treatment for herpes virus infection showed dramatic improvement.

Research Funding Low for Chronic Fatigue Syndrome

According to the Centers for Disease Control and Prevention, chronic fatigue syndrome can be as disabling as multiple sclerosis, lupus, rheumatoid arthritis, heart disease, and chronic obstructive pulmonary disease—but as this graph shows, those illnesses receive significantly more funding from the National Institutes of Health than is allocated toward CFS.

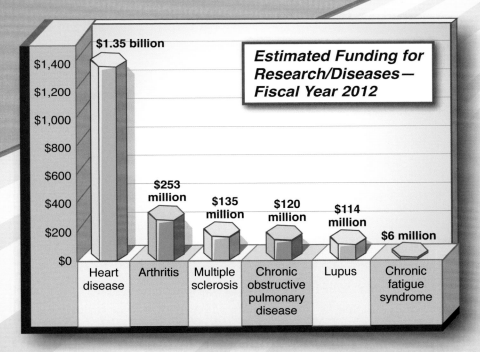

Estimated Funding for Research/Diseases— Fiscal Year 2012

Source: National Institutes of Health, "Estimates of Funding for Various Research, Conditions, and Disease Categories (RCDC)," March 15, 2011. http://report.nih.gov.

- According to the Mayo Clinic, treatments that involve medications intended to boost the immune system's **ability to fight infection** have not proved to be consistently effective in CFS sufferers, and some patients have experienced severe side effects.

Key People and Advocacy Groups

Sir Donald Acheson: A British physician who coined the term *benign myalgic encephalomyelitis* in 1955 to describe the mysterious illness that later became known in the United States as chronic fatigue syndrome.

George Miller Beard: A New York City neurologist who identified a mysterious ailment that he called neurasthenia, which caused profound exhaustion, headaches, insomnia, noises in the ear, and other symptoms much like what is now known as chronic fatigue syndrome.

David S. Bell: A general medicine physician from Lyndonville, New York, who treated a large number of patients with CFS in what became known as the Lyndonville cluster.

Rich Carson: A former long-distance runner who was stricken with CFS in 1981 and who founded the group ProHealth. In 2006 Carson launched the Campaign for a Fair Name in an effort to change the name *chronic fatigue syndrome*, which he believes trivializes the seriousness of the illness.

Paul R. Cheney: One of two physicians who treated patients during the 1984 CFS epidemic in Incline Village, Nevada; he went on to pioneer clinical research and become known as an internationally recognized expert on the illness.

Alan Goldberg: Stricken with CFS in 1985, Goldberg cofounded the CFIDS Association of America in Charlotte, North Carolina, in 1987.

Seymour Grufferman: An immunologist who proposed the term *chronic fatigue and immune dysfunction syndrome* to reflect the immune abnormalities characteristic of the disease, as well as to prevent *fatigue* from being the key feature of its name.

Walter Gunn: The principal CFS investigator for the CDC who became known as a whistle-blower for bringing public attention to his colleagues' misappropriation of money provided by Congress to study the disease.

Laura Hillenbrand: The author of the books *Seabiscuit* and *Unbroken*, Hillenbrand has suffered from CFS since she was 19 years old.

Marc Iverson: Originally misdiagnosed with Epstein-Barr virus infection, Iverson cofounded the CFIDS Association of America in 1987 and served as the organization's president until his resignation in 2001.

Carol Jessop: A San Francisco physician who became known as a pioneer in CFS research and was often quoted in medical literature because of her large caseload of CFS patients.

Nancy Kaiser: A woman from Albuquerque, New Mexico, who suffered from one of the most severe cases of CFS that doctors had ever seen. After being sick for 10 years, Kaiser became "Patient 00," the first CFS sufferer to receive the experimental AIDS drug Ampligen.

Jose G. Montoya: A Stanford School of Medicine professor who specializes in infectious disease and is a recognized authority on CFS.

Daniel L. Peterson: One of two physicians who treated patients during the 1984 CFS epidemic in Incline Village, Nevada; he became known as a pioneer in treatment of the illness and cofounded the Whittemore Peterson Institute for Neuro-Immune Disease at the University of Nevada.

Dorothy Wall: The author of the book *Encounters with the Invisible: Unseen Illness, Controversy, and Chronic Fatigue Syndrome*, which chronicles her own personal experience with the disease, as well as examines the perspectives of physicians, researchers, and CFS advocates.

Chronology

1869
American neurologist George Miller Beard identifies a mysterious ailment that he calls neurasthenia, which causes profound exhaustion, headaches, insomnia, noises in the ear, and other symptoms much like what later becomes known as chronic fatigue syndrome.

1948
A mysterious illness breaks out in Akureyri, Iceland, and sickens nearly 500 people. Because many patients become paralyzed, the illness is first thought to be poliomyelitis, but this proves to be incorrect. Decades later, the outbreak is determined to have been CFS.

1970
British psychiatrist Colin P. McEvedy and physician A.W. Beard publish a paper in which they claim that the reports of benign myalgic encephalomyelitis are psychosocial in nature, likely due to "mass hysteria" rather than physical ailments.

1870   1930   1950   1970

1934
An outbreak of a mysterious illness affects 10 percent of physicians and nurses at Los Angeles County Hospital. Originally believed to be poliomyelitis, the illness is later determined to have been CFS.

1985
Outbreaks of CFS are reported in Incline Village, Nevada, and Lyndonville, New York, which collectively affect more than 500 people.

1987
CFS sufferers Marc Iverson and Alan Goldberg found an advocacy organization that later becomes known as the CFIDS Association of America.

1956
The British journal the *Lancet* publishes an editorial called "A New Clinical Entity?" in which *benign myalgic encephalomyelitis* is suggested as the acceptable name for an illness that involves extreme fatigue and severe flu-like symptoms.

1988
The CDC selects the name *chronic fatigue syndrome* and publishes its case definition in the *Annals of Internal Medicine*.

Chronology

1990

A clinical trial in which severely debilitated CFS patients are treated twice weekly with the experimental AIDS drug Ampligen finds evidence of significantly improved physical function, increased activity, and enhanced cognitive ability.

2010

Australia, Canada, New Zealand, and Britain ban people with a history of CFS from donating blood; later the same year the American Red Cross bans blood donations from people with a history of the illness.

1991

Philadelphia virologist Elaine DeFreitas finds retroviral DNA in 24 of 30 CFS patients, which suggests that the illness could be associated with a retrovirus.

2003

The US Department of Health and Human Services establishes the Chronic Fatigue Syndrome Advisory Committee, which is charged with maintaining a focus on patients with CFS, working collaboratively, and focusing on an evidence- and science-based approach to research.

1990

2010

1994

The CDC issues a revised case definition for CFS that better distinguishes it from other types of unexplained fatigue and includes specific diagnostic criteria.

1996

The US Congress asks the secretary of the US Department of Health and Human Services to consider renaming CFS, but the name is not changed.

2009

A team of researchers publishes a study in the publication *Science* that links the human retrovirus XMRV with CFS. The findings are later discredited by other studies.

2005

Author Dorothy Wall publishes a book called *Encounters with the Invisible: Unseen Illness, Controversy, and Chronic Fatigue Syndrome*, which chronicles her years-long battle with CFS and examines the perspectives of researchers and physicians.

2011

A meeting of the Chronic Fatigue Syndrome Advisory Committee is held in Washington, DC; numerous CFS sufferers and patient advocates present testimony, imploring the government for more funding and a greater emphasis on research to find the cause.

Related Organizations

Centers for Disease Control and Prevention (CDC)

1600 Clifton Rd.
Atlanta, GA 30333
phone: (800) 232-4636
e-mail: cdcinfo@cdc.gov • website: www.cdc.gov

The CDC is dedicated to protecting health and promoting quality of life through the prevention and control of disease, injury, and disability. Its website's Chronic Fatigue Syndrome section offers news articles, information sheets, and a variety of related publications.

CFIDS Association of America

PO Box 220398
Charlotte, NC 28222-0398
phone: (704) 365-2343
e-mail: cfids@cfids.org • website: www.cfids.org

The CFIDS Association of America is a charitable organization dedicated to ending the pain, suffering, and disability caused by CFS. Its website offers research information, the *SolveCFS* publication, CFSID*Link* newsletter, and an "About CFS" section with general information about CFS.

International Association for Chronic Fatigue Syndrome/ Myalgic Encephalopathy (CFS/ME)

27 N. Wacker Dr., Suite 416
Chicago, IL 60606
phone: (847) 258-7248 • fax: (847) 579-0975
e-mail: admin@iacfsme.org • website: www.iacfsme.org

The International Association for CFS/ME is dedicated to research, education, treatment, and finding a cure for CFS/ME. Its website offers a newsletter, fact sheets, archived quarterly bulletins, research information, and abstracts of articles.

Mayo Clinic

200 First St. SW
Rochester, MN 55905
phone: (507) 284-2511 • fax: (507) 284-0161
website: www.mayoclinic.com

The Mayo Clinic is a world-renowned medical facility that is dedicated to patient care, education, and research. Its website offers information about CFS symptoms, risk factors, causes, treatment, lifestyle, and home remedies.

ME Association

7 Apollo Office Ct.
Radclive Rd.
Gawcott
Buckingham MK18 4DF, UK
phone: +44 (0)1280 827070
e-mail: meconnect@meassociation.org.uk
website: www.meassociation.org.uk

The ME Association funds and supports research, education, and training, as well as provides information and support to people in the United Kingdom who are affected by ME/CFS. Its website features research updates, the *ME Essentials* magazine, and fact sheets that cover the disease's effects, causes, treatment, and prognosis.

ME Research UK

Gateway, N. Methven St.
Perth PH1 5PP, UK
phone: +44 (0)1738 451234
e-mail: meruk@pkavs.org.uk • website: www.meresearch.org.uk

The ME Research UK's principal goal is to commission and fund scientific research into the causes, consequences, and treatment of ME/CFS. Its website offers numerous informative publications, research papers, articles, and the *Breakthrough* magazine.

National Alliance for Myalgic Encephalomyelitis (NAME)

website: www.name-us.org

NAME is an organization that believes ME is a specific neurological disease that is not accurately conveyed by the term *chronic fatigue syndrome*. Its website offers numerous publications, news articles, and research information.

National Chronic Fatigue and Immune Dysfunction Syndrome (CFIDS) Foundation

103 Aletha Rd.
Needham, MA 02492
phone: (781) 449-3535 • fax: (781) 449-8606
e-mail: info@ncf-net.org • website: www.ncf-net.org

The National CFIDS Foundation funds medical research for CFS, as well as provides information, education, and support to people who suffer from it. Its website offers an archived newsletter, a variety of articles, and other resources.

National Chronic Fatigue Syndrome and Fibromyalgia Association (NCFSFA)

PO Box 18426
Kansas City, MO 64133
phone: (816) 737-1343 • fax: (816) 524-6782
e-mail: information@ncfsfa.org • website: www.ncfsfa.org

The NCFSFA seeks to educate and inform the public, patients and their families, and health professionals about the nature and impact of CFS. Its website offers frequently asked questions, information tailored for patients and physicians, a "Suicide Is Not an Option" publication, and articles about a wide variety of topics.

National Institutes of Health Genetic and Rare Diseases Center

Genetic and Rare Diseases Information Center
PO Box 8126
Gaithersburg, MD 20898-8126
phone: (301) 251-4925 • fax: (301) 251-4911
website: http://rarediseases.info.nih.gov

The Genetic and Rare Diseases Center exists to help people find useful information about genetic and rare diseases. Its website serves as a portal to a broad range of information about rare diseases, including definitions, causes, and treatments, and the site's search engine produces a number of articles specifically about CFS.

National Myalgic Encephalomyelitis/Fibromyalgia (ME/FM) Action Network

512, 33 Banner Rd.
Nepean, ON K2H 8V7 Canada
phone: (613) 829-6667 • fax: (613) 829-8518
e-mail: mefmaction@ncf.ca • website: www.mefmaction.com

The ME/FM Action Network is a Canadian charitable organization that provides support, advocacy, education, and research on ME/FM. Its website offers news articles, the *Quest* quarterly newsletter, a Youth Corner, legal issue publications, videos, and podcasts.

ProHealth

2040 Alameda Padre Serra
Santa Barbara, CA 93103
phone: (800) 366-6056 • fax: (805) 965-0042
website: www.prohealth.com

Founded by CFS sufferer Rich Carson, ProHealth is dedicated to proactive health management. Its website offers research and treatment news, interviews and live chats with physicians, information about traditional and alternative treatments, and the monthly newsletter *Healthwatch*, as well as a searchable library of articles on numerous topics.

For Further Research

Books

Michael Andersen and Michael Woo, *My Physician Guide to Chronic Fatigue Syndrome*. Charleston, SC: CreateSpace, 2011.

Sylvia Engdahl, *Chronic Fatigue Syndrome*. Farmington Hills, MI: Greenhaven, 2011.

Chantal K. Hoey-Sanders, *I Have Fibromyalgia/Chronic Fatigue Syndrome, but It Doesn't Have Me!,* Bloomington, IN: Balboa, 2011.

Michael E. Hyland, *The Origins of Health and Disease*. Cambridge: Cambridge University Press, 2011.

Elliot Jacob, ed., *Medifocus Guidebook On: Chronic Fatigue Syndrome*. Charleston, SC: CreateSpace, 2011.

Pam Kidd, *I Have CFS but I Don't Look Sick*. Frederick, MD: PublishAmerica, 2011.

Eva Svoboda and Kristof Zelenjcik, *Chronic Fatigue Syndrome: Symptoms, Causes and Prevention*. Hauppauge, NY: Nova Science, 2010.

Periodicals

Ewen Callaway, "Fighting for a Cause," *Nature*, March 17, 2011.

Denise Grady, "Virus Is Found in Many with Chronic Fatigue Syndrome," *New York Times*, October 8, 2009.

Leonard A. Jason, "An Illness That's Hard to Live with—or Define," *Wall Street Journal*, March 5, 2011.

Hillary Johnson, "A Case of Chronic Denial," *New York Times*, October 21, 2009.

Claudia Kalb, "Validation in a Virus?," *Newsweek*, December 6, 2010.

Amy Dockser Marcus, "Amid War on a Mystery Disease, Patients Clash with Scientists," *Wall Street Journal*, March 12, 2011.

———, "The Puzzle of Chronic Fatigue," *Wall Street Journal*, March 5, 2011.

Amie Ninh, "Chronic Fatigue in Teens: Rare but Serious," *Time*, April 18, 2011.

Nathan Seppa, "Body & Brain: Pathogen Fingered as a Potential Culprit in Chronic Fatigue Syndrome: Little-Known Retrovirus Found in Many People with Condition," *Science News*, December 9, 2009.

Rob Stein, "Chronic Fatigue Patients Barred from Blood Donation," *Washington Post*, December 3, 2010.

Trine Tsouderos, "Hope Outrunning Science on Chronic Fatigue Syndrome," *Chicago Tribune*, June 7, 2010.

David Tuller, "Defining an Illness Is Fodder for Debate," *New York Times*, March 4, 2011.

Brian Vastag, "Mouse Virus Doesn't Cause Chronic Fatigue Syndrome," *Washington Post*, May 31, 2011.

Women's Health Updates, "Chronic Fatigue Syndrome," December 2010.

Internet Sources

Centers for Disease Control and Prevention, "Chronic Fatigue Syndrome," March 24, 2011. www.cdc.gov/cfs/index.html.

John Falk, "Chronic Fatigue Syndrome and Psychotherapy," *Huffington Post*, March 1, 2011. www.huffingtonpost.com/john-falk/chronic-fatigue-syndrome-_b_829651.html.

J. Carlton Gartner Jr., "Chronic Fatigue Syndrome," KidsHealth, July 2010. http://kidshealth.org/parent/system/ill/cfs.html.

Mayo Clinic, "Chronic Fatigue Syndrome," June 19, 2009. www.mayoclinic.com/health/chronic-fatigue-syndrome/DS00395.

National Institutes of Health, "Chronic Fatigue Syndrome," February 7, 2010. www.nlm.nih.gov/medlineplus/ency/article/001244.htm.

New York Times Health Guide, "Chronic Fatigue Syndrome," February 3, 2009. http://health.nytimes.com/health/guides/disease/chronic-fatigue-syndrome/overview.html.

Tara Parker-Pope, "An Author Escapes from Chronic Fatigue Syndrome," *Well* (blog), *New York Times*, February 4, 2011. http://well.blogs.nytimes.com/2011/02/04/an-author-escapes-from-chronic-fatigue-syndrome.

Source Notes

Overview

1. Molly Billings, "Unlocking Chronic Fatigue Syndrome," *Wall Street Journal*, March 22, 2011. http://online.wsj.com.
2. Billings, "Unlocking Chronic Fatigue Syndrome."
3. Quoted in Tara Parker-Pope, "An Author Escapes from Chronic Fatigue Syndrome," *Well* (blog), *New York Times*, February 4, 2011. well.blogs.nytimes.com.
4. CFIDS Association of America, "Prevalence: How Many People Have CFS?," 2011. www.cfids.org.
5. Alison McCook, "Chronic Fatigue Rare but Serious in Teens," Reuters, April 18, 2011. www.reuters.com.
6. Mayo Clinic, "Chronic Fatigue Syndrome," June 19, 2009. www.mayoclinic.com.
7. Laurel Bertrand, "My Story," *Dreams at Stake*, May 25, 2009. http://dreamsatstake.blogspot.com.
8. Bertrand, "My Story."
9. B. Sigurdsson, J. Sigurjonsson, J.H.J. Sigurdsson, J. Thorkelsson, K.R. Gudmundsson, "A Disease Epidemic in Iceland Simulating Poliomyelitis," *American Journal of Hygiene*, April 13, 1950, p. 222.
10. Centers for Disease Control and Prevention, "Chronic Fatigue Syndrome," March 24, 2011. http://www.cdc.gov.
11. University of Maryland Medical Center, "Chronic Fatigue Syndrome—Causes," January 13, 2009. www.umm.edu.
12. Leonard A. Jason, "An Illness That's Hard to Live with—or Define," *Wall Street Journal*, March 5, 2011. http://online.wsj.com.
13. David S. Bell, *The Doctor's Guide to Chronic Fatigue Syndrome*. Reading, MA: Addison-Wesley, 1994, pp. 222–23.
14. Centers for Disease Control and Prevention, "Chronic Fatigue Syndrome."
15. Bertrand, "My Story."
16. Hillary Johnson, "A Case of Chronic Denial," *New York Times*, October 20, 2009. www.nytimes.com.
17. Alexis Cairns, "In the Dark," *The Corner Room* (blog), December 8, 2010. http://thecornerroom.tumblr.com.
18. Cairns, "In the Dark."
19. Centers for Disease Control and Prevention, "Chronic Fatigue Syndrome."
20. Johnson, "A Case of Chronic Denial."
21. Johnson, "A Case of Chronic Denial."
22. Mayo Clinic, "Chronic Fatigue Syndrome."
23. Billings, "Unlocking Chronic Fatigue Syndrome."

What Is Chronic Fatigue Syndrome?

24. Mindy Kitei, "Have You No Sense of Decency?," CFS Central, May 11, 2011. www.cfscentral.com.
25. Kitei, "Have You No Sense of Decency?"
26. George Miller Beard, "Neurasthenia, or Nervous Exhaustion," *Boston Medical and Surgical Journal*, April 29, 1869, p. 208.
27. *Lancet*, "A New Clinical Entity?," editorial, May 26, 1956. www.meresearch.org.uk.
28. Karen Lee Richards, "A Disease in Search of a Name," ProHealth, January 3, 2007. www.prohealth.com.
29. Quoted in Karen Lee Richards, "Meet Rich Carson, Patient and ME/CFS & FM Fundraiser—and Learn How Pro-

Health Began," A Fair Name, 2006. www.afairname.org.

30. Richards, "A Disease in Search of a Name."

31. Dov Michaeli, "The Puzzle of Chronic Fatigue Syndrome," *The Doctor Weighs In* (blog), February 21, 2011. www.thedoctorweighsin.com.

32. Michaeli, "The Puzzle of Chronic Fatigue Syndrome."

33. Quoted in Kristy Katzmann, "Dr. David S. Bell, MD—Dedicated to the Plight of Chronic Fatigue Syndrome Patients Since 1985," ProHealth, September 4, 2007. www.prohealth.com.

34. Quoted in Katzmann, "Dr. David S. Bell, MD—Dedicated to the Plight of Chronic Fatigue Syndrome Patients Since 1985."

35. James P. Terry, "Gulf War Syndrome: Addressing Undiagnosed Illnesses from the First War with Iraq," *Veterans Law Review*, 2009. www.bva.va.gov.

36. Terry, "Gulf War Syndrome."

37. CFIDS Association of America, "Fiscal Year 2011 Appropriations Requests: Department of Defense," 2010. www.cfids.org.

38. Quoted in Joan Livingston, "25 Year Follow-Up in Chronic Fatigue Syndrome: Rising Incapacity," Massachusetts CFIDS/ME & FM Association, April 16, 2011. www.masscfids.org.

What Causes Chronic Fatigue Syndrome?

39. University of Maryland Medical Center, "Chronic Fatigue Syndrome—Causes."

40. University of Maryland Medical Center, "Chronic Fatigue Syndrome—Causes."

41. Dedra Buchwald et al., "A Chronic Illness Characterized by Fatigue, Neurologic and Immunologic Disorders, and Active Human Herpesvirus Type 6 Infection," *Annals of Internal Medicine*, January 15, 1992. www.cfsuntied.com.

42. Robert H. Shmerling, "Chronic Fatigue Syndrome: Names and Claims," Aetna InteliHealth, May 26, 2009. www.intelihealth.com.

43. Stanford School of Medicine, "What Is Infection-Associated Chronic Fatigue Syndrome?," 2011. http://chronicfatigue.stanford.edu.

44. Stanford School of Medicine, "What Is Infection-Associated Chronic Fatigue Syndrome?"

45. Shmerling, "Chronic Fatigue Syndrome."

46. Centers for Disease Control and Prevention, "Epstein-Barr Virus and Infectious Mononucleosis," May 16, 2006. www.cdc.gov.

47. Ben Z. Katz et al., "Chronic Fatigue Syndrome After Infectious Mononucleosis in Adolescents," *Pediatrics*, July 2009. http://pediatrics.aappublications.org.

48. Quoted in Denise Grady, "Is a Virus the Cause of Chronic Fatigue Syndrome?," *New York Times*, October 12, 2009. www.nytimes.com.

49. Wellcome Trust Sanger Institute, "Chronic Fatigue Syndrome Is Not Caused by XMRV," December 20, 2010. www.sanger.ac.uk.

50. Quoted in Jon Cohen, "New Data Spark Retraction Request for Chronic Fatigue Virus Study," *Science Now*, May 31, 2011. http://news.sciencemag.org.

51. Bruce Alberts, "Editorial Expression of Concern," *Science*, June 1, 2011. www.sciencemag.org.

What Are the Effects of Chronic Fatigue Syndrome?

52. Quoted in Jennifer Johnson, "Local Man Battles Chronic Fatigue Syn-

drome," 13WHAM News, May 13, 2011. www.13wham.com.

53. Quoted in Johnson, "Local Man Battles Chronic Fatigue Syndrome."

54. Billings, "Unlocking Chronic Fatigue Syndrome."

55. Lindsey Dunlap, testimony before the US Department of Health and Human Services Chronic Fatigue Syndrome Advisory Committee, May 11, 2011. www.hhs.gov.

56. John Falk, "Chronic Fatigue Syndrome and Psychotherapy," *Huffington Post*, March 1, 2011. www.huffingtonpost.com.

57. Falk, "Chronic Fatigue Syndrome and Psychotherapy."

58. Toni Bernhard, "The Stigma of Chronic Fatigue Syndrome," *Turning Straw into Gold* (blog), *Psychology Today*, April 20, 2011. www.psychologytoday.com.

59. Bernhard, "The Stigma of Chronic Fatigue Syndrome."

60. Bernhard, "The Stigma of Chronic Fatigue Syndrome."

61. Bertrand, "My Story."

62. Bertrand, "My Story."

63. University of Maryland Medical Center, "Chronic Fatigue Syndrome—Prognosis," January 13, 2009. www.umm.edu.

64. Quoted in McCook, "Chronic Fatigue Rare but Serious in Teens."

65. Bertrand, "My Story."

Can People Overcome Chronic Fatigue Syndrome?

66. University of Maryland Medical Center, "Chronic Fatigue Syndrome—Introduction."

67. Centers for Disease Control and Prevention, "Chronic Fatigue Syndrome."

68. Robert Gonzalez, "Recovering from Chronic Fatigue Syndrome," *One Man's Voice* (blog), May 19, 2011. www.robert-gonzalez.com.

69. Gonzalez, "Recovering from Chronic Fatigue Syndrome."

70. Gonzalez, "Recovering from Chronic Fatigue Syndrome."

71. Gonzalez, "Recovering from Chronic Fatigue Syndrome."

72. Gonzalez, "Recovering from Chronic Fatigue Syndrome."

73. Quoted in Richard Knox, "Psychotherapy and Exercise Look Best to Treat Chronic Fatigue Syndrome," National Public Radio, February 18, 2011. www.npr.org.

74. Robert J. Hedaya, "Chronic Fatigue Syndrome," *Health Matters* (blog), *Psychology Today*, February 23, 2010. www.psychologytoday.com.

75. Falk, "Chronic Fatigue Syndrome and Psychotherapy."

76. Quoted in Knox, "Psychotherapy and Exercise Look Best to Treat Chronic Fatigue Syndrome."

77. Quoted in Knox, "Psychotherapy and Exercise Look Best to Treat Chronic Fatigue Syndrome."

78. Quoted in Parker-Pope, "An Author Escapes from Chronic Fatigue Syndrome."

79. Quoted in Parker-Pope, "An Author Escapes from Chronic Fatigue Syndrome."

80. Quoted in Parker-Pope, "An Author Escapes from Chronic Fatigue Syndrome."

81. Bertrand, "My Story."

List of Illustrations

Index

About the Author

Peggy J. Parks holds a bachelor of science degree from Aquinas College in Grand Rapids, Michigan, where she graduated magna cum laude. An author who has written more than 100 educational books for children and young adults, Parks lives in Muskegon, Michigan, a town that she says inspires her writing because of its location on the shores of Lake Michigan.